Also by Joyce Wadler

My Breast: One Woman's Cancer Story

Liaison

Cured

My Ovarian Cancer Story

by

Joyce Wadler

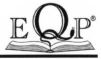

E-QUALITY PRESS

CURED
An E-QUALITY PRESS production / June 2013
UUID# DC22C920-AAA1-11E2-9E96-0800200C9A66

Originally published as a serial in *New York* Magazine,
September, 1997

An E-QUALITY PRESS book

The name E-QUALITY PRESS and its logo, consisting of
the letters "EQP" over an open book with power cord, are
registered trademarks of E-QUALITY PRESS.
www.e-qualitypress.com

PRODUCED IN THE UNITED STATES OF AMERICA

In Memory Of Heidi Handman

CONTENTS

Foreword

WHEN I WAS DIAGNOSED with advanced ovarian cancer, 15 years ago, well meaning friends told me to buy comedian Gilda Radner's book about her experience with the disease. It was very inspirational, they said.

There was one problem with this suggestion: Gilda Radner had died of ovarian cancer.

I did not. My ovarian cancer was cured and I returned to a healthy, normal life: I became a reporter at *The New York Times* where I worked for 15 years; I went on bike trips in France and Northern California; I had love affairs—nice, normal, sexually satisfying love affairs.

I also learned something very important: Things are always changing in Cancer World. When Gilda Radner, whose cancer was more advanced than mine when it was found, was diagnosed in 1986, drugs and treatments with which I was treated when I was diagnosed in 1995, were not available to her.

Nor was anything known about the BRCA-1 genetic mutation, which gives a woman a higher risk of developing breast and ovarian cancer, and which, it turned out, I carry.

When I first published my story in *New York* Magazine several years ago there were those who felt it was best not to know if you carry this mutation. They were wrong. If you know you have the BRCA-1 or BRCA-2 mutations you can take steps to prevent ovarian cancer or catch it early. I'll have more about that at the end of this book. For now, here's my story.

And remember: People can be cured.

I

WHEN I WAS A KID and knew everything there was to know in the universe, I had an ongoing argument with my grandmother. She had hot-footed it out of Russia around 1910—it being a particularly bad place for a Jew—and she still held on to what I believed to be the old-country view: Stash your money in your brassiere and keep one eye on the exit, because our lives are governed by dark and uncontrollable forces and if something can go wrong, it will. "You should only be lucky," she said.

"This is America, Gram," I'd say. "You make your own luck."

Now, however, having had both breast and ovarian cancer in five years, and having learned I am carrying one of the newly discovered genetic mutations that occur in an estimated 1 in 50 Ashkenazic Jews, I have come to respect my grandmother's point of view: It is helpful to be lucky. And I am not.

My breast cancer was caught early, but my ovarian cancer, like most ovarian cancers, was what the doctors call "advanced." Despite my regular visits to the gynecologist, by the time the surgeon snared it, it had contentedly spread: setting up a number of little encampments on the omentum, the fatty apron of tissue that falls off the stomach and drapes over the transverse colon; twisting around the large intestine; gluing the uterus to the colon. My chance of surviving four years from the time of my diagnosis is 50 percent. Two years after my diagnosis I have no way of knowing whether I am cured or the cancer will come back.

Years of newspaper work have taught me the importance of a snazzy tag for disasters, so I have named me: Middle-aged Mutant Jewish Writer. I looked after my health and it still didn't matter. I was my own Unabomber, carrying my future from the time I was born, caught in a genetic accident. If the test for 185delAG had been around a few years earlier, if I'd known my true medical genealogy, if there were routine screening for ovarian cancer, I might be feeling better.

"Is there anything else that comes with this gene?" I ask my doctor. "A house in the country? A car? A guy? You know, I could really use a guy."

"Nope, you got it all," he says.

II

THIS IS WHAT MIDDLE-AGED mutant Jewish writer, growing up in a boardinghouse in the Catskills, knew of her. family: That her maternal my grandfather, Max Aronowitz, came from Romania and entered the country informally, through Canada. That her maternal grandmother, Gussie Tauber, claimed to be from Vienna but was not. That there were, on my mother's side, endless configurations of cousins, and when they were young, the girls were wild.

The wild Aronowitz women: My mother, Milly, runs away to Miami at 17, getting a job painting flamingos on glass. Her favorite niece, Gorgeous Roberta, has so many boyfriends that my mother, now married and respectable, stops speaking to her for a while. Roberta's daughter, Sophie, makes the family proud by becoming a Miss Israel, then scandalizes them by posing naked in one of the tabloids and discussing what great sex she has with her boyfriend.

"*RRRRIIIIIPPPPPP!*" A sound like thunder as pictures of Sophie are ripped from Aronowitz refrigerators around the world and torn apart.

"How could she do it?" Ma asks. Which astonishes me. Even before I have emerged as Mutant Middle-aged Jewish Writer, I get it: It's in her genes, I think. She's a flaming Jewish sexpot Let them find a cure for that.

But no cancer. Nowhere, among Ma and her mother and her sister and her half-brothers and her cousins and her nieces, is there any cancer.

There is no breast or ovarian cancer on my father's side, either. My grandmother, Gussie, does have one sister who dies of pancreatic cancer; but that is one in five. My grandmother makes it, cancer-free, to her late eighties, as does my mother's mother.

It is true that if there were cancer, they might not discuss it, because there is a big tradition of not upsetting the children. There are, in her heavy, dark photo albums, a lot of people my grandmother doesn't want to discuss. The nephew who had polio and committed suicide. The guy on a country road in Poland, wearing a jacket and pants that are too small, staring anxiously at the camera as if it were an alien form, which it probably is.

"Who's that?" I ask.

She turns the pages fast.

"Europe," she says. "Gone."

Or, sometimes, one word: "Hitler."

I grow up and come to the Village, making a living working for newspapers and magazines. In romance, my grandmother would say, I am not lucky; at 47, when this adventure begins, I have not even managed a first marriage. But I have had my friends for years.

My best friend is Herb, a comedy writer, whom I met twenty years ago when we were reporters at the old New York *Post*. I looked across the city room and there he was, a tall, thin, bearded guy with a nice smile. We tried it romantically for a while, but it did not work. In most other ways, however, we fit: Visiting friends in Africa who are correspondents for the L.A. *Times,* we both decline when they hear about a massacre in Somalia and want me and Herb, obvious tourists, to come with them "as cover" to check it out.

"You're kidding, right?" I say.

"We're the feature people, remember?" says Herb. "We do the jokes."

My closest old boyfriend is Donal. He is a photographer, a big, handsome man with a honey-colored mustache, the quietest guy in our crowd and the best educated. We lived together, on and off, for six. years. Unlike some of the other men I dated, Donal didn't have any problem with Herb. The problem was, Donal had no head for business and he was always in the darkroom, and when he was not, he was late. Also, he was the worst housekeeper in the world. We break up. A few years later, in the summer of '91, Donal tells me he has become gay. Herb and I are stunned.

"Did you see this coming?" asks Herb. "I didn't see this coming. Aren't gay men supposed to be neat?"

Also: "Only Donal would pick a time like this to become gay."

When we go to a photo exhibit where Donal and his boyfriend are expected to be, I am tense.

"What do you think he'll look like?" I ask Herb.

"A lot like you, I would think," Herb says.

I do not meet the boyfriend at the exhibit. I meet him a few months later, at St. Vincents, in the HIV ward. He had been tested; he wasn't supposed to get sick. Two years later, the boyfriend, whose name is Rick, is dead, and Donal is positive.

But I am lucky. Donal's change of life happens well after we are broken up—the first thing Don wants me to know is that my health was never at risk.

My luck holds even when I get breast cancer, at 43. The cancer is encapsulated, so that I can be treated with lumpectomy and not lose a breast. When I have chemotherapy, it is a sort that does not make me lose my hair or exhaust me. Chemo Lite. It takes five months, and during that time I work out, go to France, and write a book about breast cancer, then a television movie. Meredith Baxter is me. I know it's lost a little of the essence when I go up to Toronto, where they're filming, and meet the guy who plays Herb.

"You mean she's a *Jewish girl?*" he says.

When the trailers show Meredith learning the lump in her breast is malignant and getting very upset, I call Ma, so she won't be upset also.

"I just want you to know, when I found out, I didn't *geschrei* like that," I tell Ma. "But you *could* have," Ma says. "And who knows? Maybe her way was better." I get off the phone. "This is so weird," I tell Herb. "I'm having sibling rivalry with a television character." "Don't think of it as television," says Herb. "Think of it as your gentile self."

I am not one of those people who live in fear of recurrence, either. Cancer has already come to the family—my father died of prostate cancer at 67 but I consider my breast cancer an aberration and do not expect to ever get sick again.

"Cancer is not a death sentence," I say when I speak to women's groups. But because I've heard the stats, that women who've had breast cancer have a higher risk of getting breast and ovarian cancer, I try to take very good care of myself.

I see my surgeon and oncologist at Memorial Sloan-Kettering every six months and have blood screens and breast exams. I see a gynecologist, outside Memorial, every six months. I like my gynecologist. He is warm; he is easy to talk to; he teaches at a university; he writes books. "So what did you get for the paperback?" he asks when I am in the stirrups.

When I have unusual vaginal bleeding, similar to a very heavy period, two years after breast cancer, after chemotherapy has put me into early menopause, my gynecologist does an endometrial biopsy—you should always check out unusual bleeding, he says. When I have chronic constipation a year later, I go to a proctologist. Neither doctor finds any problems. The gynecologist, in fact, says I'm in great shape.

"If you didn't tell me you were in menopause, I couldn't tell," he says.

A milestone, I think—my first middle-age compliment. There is another reason I don't worry about cancer: I have the best doctor on the block. His name is Larry Norton; he is the chief of breast-cancer medicine at Memorial Sloan-Kettering, and in addition to being the son of a newspaper guy, which is the best lineage I feel anyone can have, and having no use for authority, he is funny and loose and smart. Also, he is obsessed. I check in with him before speaking about breast cancer, to make sure I'm up to date, and he is always in the shop.

"Don't you have a family?" I say, eight o'clock Friday night, cramming for an October lecture. "Don't you ever stop?"

He talks fast, a real New Yorker, which is another thing I like.

"I *love* my family," he says. "I *love* my kids. But you ask me what their favorite candy bar is, what movies they like, I couldn't tell you. My wife could tell you; I couldn't tell you. You know why I can't stop? I'll tell you a story."

A writer on the way to the bathroom will stop for a story. I settle in.

"You ever talk to a crowd and you see somebody who doesn't seem to belong there?" Norton says. "This happened to me once. I'm somewhere in the Midwest, a medical thing, I see this couple; they just don't fit. I give this talk, very technical; afterwards, somebody brings them over. It turns out a few years ago she had inflammatory breast cancer. She goes to her doctor. He says, 'I believe what you have is very serious, but I just read a paper by this doctor in New York'—I'm the doctor in New York—'and he's got a way to treat this.' So these people, I think they're farmers, have driven a hundred miles, paid $300 for a lecture they've understood maybe three words of and a meal you could not eat, just to shake my hand and thank me for saving her life."

He sounds like he is choking up.

I feel safe with Norton. Beyond safe. I feel smug.

That is where I am when this story begins, in the fall of '95: Smug City.

My love life, it is true, is not so hot. I have not had a real boyfriend in more than four years, when I dated a charming but troublesome newspaper guy named Nick DeStefano, and it eats at me. It is the reason I keep a stack of books by my bed and hate

Sundays. I feel incomplete and lonely without someone in my life, and the old make-do solution, spending the night with a good male friend, is less feasible these days.

"So whaddaya say we go to the country and lock ourselves in a room for a weekend?" I ask Izz, the left-wing lawyer, a boyfriend in the days when Abbie Hoffman was underground.

"You confuse me with the Italian Stallion," says Izz, who is 58. "I'm an old Jew. I run for the curb, I get winded."

I am also having some minor physical problems. Constipation is still bothering me. I've had another instance of vaginal spotting, which I'm scheduled to have checked out, as well as what the gynecologist's nurse calls a "slightly irregular" Pap smear. I have a bad feeling when I hear that. Just before I was diagnosed with breast cancer, a doctor aspirated a lump in my breast and told me some cells were "slightly" abnormal. Ten days later, he took a tumor the size of a robin's egg out of my breast. But the nurse had been insistent: "Barely noticeable." "Probably an infection." "We'll give you a prescription for sulfa cream and redo the Pap in six weeks."

But overall, I'm feeling good.

I have just had my six-month checkup with Norton, and he's said what all my doctors say: "You're healthy." I've just finished some work in a new line—television—a script about a teenage-girl detective, which everybody loves, which means they will change every word in it. In newspaper work, this used to make me crazy. In this case, I don't mind. I like the people I am working with, and, even more, I like a story where I can ensure happy endings.

Reality, lately, has been bringing me down. Donal has been HIV-positive now for two years. I try not to think about this, that Donal, who is almost like an ex-husband, has something inside him that will kill him. And though I am not generally good at repression, sometimes it works: Donal is a big, strong man; he carries 40 pounds of photo equipment, he is not sick. Often, I forget.

"You know," I tell him one day in August, when we're eating ice cream and strolling around the neighborhood, "it's sometimes hard for me to remember I had cancer."

"That's the difference between us," he says. "Every day that passes, you're further away from the thing and I'm closer."

Make-believe is easier, and I'm about to head up to Nickelodeon and meet the teenage actress who will be the star of the new show, when the phone rings.

It's Rory, Larry Norton's nurse.

I am so smug, I don't even get nervous.

"Your blood tests—one was a little high, so we'd like you to come back and redo it," she says, a little too casual.

I'm so smug, I've never paid any attention to those tests.

"What blood test?" I ask.

"Your CA 15-3." she says. "Just slightly. The other one, your CEA, is normal."

I'm starting to get a bad feeling here—that word *slightly* again. I am also confused. I grab the nearest piece of paper I can find to write it down and get it straight: CEA is a screen for certain types of cancer like breast and colon; CA 15-3 is the breast-cancer marker. Normal CA 15-3, says Rory, in answer to my question, is anything between 0 and 36.

And mine is?

"Seventy" she says. "That might sound high, but we have people whose markers are in the thousands. A lot of things can make it high. Pregnancy, fibroids . . . things we don't know."

I am definitely not pregnant. I have never had fibroids.

"What was my last marker?" I ask.

"Seventeen, on April 4, 1995," she says, and I can hear the reluctance in her voice.

"Before that?"

"Ten," she says.

Four hours later, having interviewed the actress on automatic pilot, I'm outside Nickelodeon, at Broadway and 44th, frantically trying to get a taxi. It's been four and a half years since I found a lump in my breast and went tearing off to a specialist, and I am struck by the similarity of the reaction. Just like before, I have turned into Zorba the Greek *I want to live!* The sky is beautiful, the bicycle messengers are beautiful, the garbage in the street is beautiful. Just like before, though I am predominantly atheist, I start negotiating with God. Just let me be okay, I think, and I'll never whine about the little things again. Just let me be okay, and I'll appreciate everything I've got.

"How did cancer change your life?" reporters used to ask me, after breast cancer.

"I buy things faster," I'd say.

But not always.

I have always loved sports cars; there was a notice of a silver Miata for sale at my gym just last week. I looked at the photo a long time, but I would never own a car in New. York. It's the Wadler in me. I see my father in Jewish Heaven, hollering, *"Piss* your money away!!!"* he yells. A car in New York is an impractical luxury. Now I make Vow One: Get me out of this mess, Great Jewish Deity, and I'll get a Miata. I'll *buy,* not lease.

By the time I get to the Breast Cancer Center, three blocks south of the main hospital on 64th, I'm manic with fear. I have some blood drawn, then go to find Norton.

He's in what looks to be a borrowed office, studying papers, and though we are the same age, he looks gray, like he has been beating down cancer all day and it has exhausted him. I hate bothering him when we don't really know that I have a problem, but at the same time, I'm petrified. I've always thought it would be nice to be Grace Kelly when stressed: cool, possibly even amused. If I had been one of those remote blonde babes, I am convinced, the Italian Stallion would have been nuts for me. But it never works. The more frightened I am, the faster I talk, and now it all comes pouring out.

"I gotta tell you, right up front, I'm not ready to die," I tell Norton.

Like he can make a call. Like he can change it.

"I mean, I'm sure you get this all the time," I say. "I know nobody comes in here saying they want to die; maybe seriously religious people don't mind it so much. To them it's probably like changing apartments. But I'm not one of those. I don't believe there's a second act. I think, when it's over, it's over."

Norton just sits there waiting, like he knows I'm not finished, which I'm not.

"I haven't had a boyfriend for *four years,*" I say.

"I knew you'd have this reaction," he says. "I told Rory it would be great if we could just sneak into your bedroom when you were sleeping and take some blood. I even thought I'd lie and tell you a vial broke. But, y'know, I never lie."

He takes a shot at a possible.

"Frequently, that assay is not accurate," he says.

"How frequently?" I ask.

"Maybe 10 percent," he says.

I do not associate these test results with my irregular bleeding or my slightly irregular Pap smear five weeks before. I don't even remember the Pap smear. I just want to know, if the numbers stay high, what we do next.

"We'd have to look carefully for the possibility of metastases," Norton says, and I decide, as he says it, that *metastases* is a lethal word, like *bullet*—that it has just become the most frightening word I know.

"I'd do a workup: CAT scan, chest, abdomen, pelvis," Norton is saying. "Likely, I wouldn't find anything. Then, in six months, something would show up. Conventionally, if you find nothing, you do nothing. But my feeling is, breast cancer is very aggressive. You treat it aggressively. We've got a very good trial here with vaccines."

Trials, to me, are what you offer people when you run out of options. I am also remembering what Dr. Susan Love said in *The Breast Book,* which is what I live by.

"Susan Love says if it's a recurrence, they can't save you," I say. "They can extend your life, but they can't save you."

I watch him mentally editing, which I can tell he's doing, because I know him as well as he knows me.

"I love Susan Love. She's a good friend, I think she's terrific," he says. "But she's a surgeon. She couldn't save your life. I could."

I go home, terrified. It's after six. Herb is off at some unknown spot, working on the "Dubious

Achievements" issue with the gang from *Esquire*. Donal, for once, is not in the darkroom. I've always known that if I ever get scared about cancer, I can call Larry Norton. But I've just talked to Larry Norton. Then I remember: The Breast Cancer Center has a psychiatric service. I get the psychologist on call. His voice is professionally soothing: crisis-control voice, I think. I see him talking down writers on the window ledge, telling them everything is all right, when he knows nothing about their lives. But crisis control works. "Do you *know* the results of the new tests?" asks the shrink. "Do you *know* the cancer has come back?" "No," I say. "Okay," he says. "Stay with that. Don't make up frightening things."

Two days later, on November 2, the results are in. In three weeks, the cancer screen has jumped from 70 to 140.

III

MUTANT MIDDLE-AGED JEWISH writer has had loads of therapy and is responsible for housing renovations in the psychiatric community from Manhattan to Fire Island. It is, in fact, how she judges her progress: When the changes on the brownstone become come more apparent than the changes in her psyche, the Mutant knows it is time to move along. In the argument of nature-vs.-nurture, she comes down firmly on the side of nurture. The family legacy she believes in, therefore, is the behavioral one.

The Mutant's mother, Milly, married into the Wadler boarding-house dynasty and drives her mother-in-law crazy by writing poems on the undersides of toilet seats: AIM STRAIGHT / WHEN YOU URINATE. Widowed for six years, 40 pounds overweight, she has three suitors following her around Daytona Beach. Her idea of a good time is riding on the back of motorcycle. She also enjoyed her time as a volunteer in the Israeli Army and would like very much for the Mutant to enlist.

The Mutant's late father, Bernie, is descended from what the Mutant's mother calls "The Worriers." When they go to the city, he worries that they've left the oven on and the house will burn down; when he goes on a trip, he gets to the airport three hours before the flight—what the Mutant has come to think of as Jewish Time.

The Mutant is an uneasy mix of the two: Her sex dreams include men in groups, but if they do not have condoms, she wakes up. And, like her father, the Mutant is a worrier. She worries when she interviews a hit man for the mob whether she is dressed properly; she worries when she sees a shrink that he will think she's a flake. Also, like her father, the Mutant has a terror of death. She does not picture it, like her mother, as an opportunity to meet God and finally have a chat with an equal She pictures it as the end.

So when the results of the new blood test come in, I'm scared.

Norton seems worried, too. He orders tests for the next day: a CAT scan in the morning, a bone scan in the afternoon. I don't ask Herb to come with me because he's up against two deadlines. But the tests frighten me. I know recurrent breast cancer can show up in any number of places—the liver, the brain. The bone scan in particular worries me: When my father had prostate cancer, it went to his bones. My mother, seeing the X-rays, called me at work. She sounded sick.

Two months later, my father was dead. Now, having the bone scan, I see the same scenario for myself: walking with a cane, maybe, or my bones splintering, too weak to hold me. The technicians aren't supposed to give you information and I am afraid to get it, but at the same time I want to know. Wanting to know wins out. *I can handle this,* I think. I play calm, so they won't think I'll flip out on them. Writer as actor. What's my motivation in this scene? Not to be dead.

"So tell me," I say, "are my bones at least attractive?" "Perfect," the tech says, and I feel my whole body relax. Whatever it is, my bones are safe.

By the time I get home, there's a message from Larry Norton. I can hear the relief in his voice. He has the results of the tests; they're "exceedingly promising."

"The bones are clean," he says when we talk later, which, thanks to being such an ace reporter, I already know. "We've got the results from the CAT scans, and they show three things: One, there's a little scar tissue on the lungs; two, there's a little nubbin on the liver, which is probably a hemangioma—"

"What's a hemangioma?" I interrupt.

"A blood vessel, nothing, we'll check it out with an MRI. Third thing—this is important—the ovaries are enlarged. *Slightly* enlarged."

He still cannot say what we are looking at, but, he says, this is good news: Whatever is wrong, we're catching it early. The ovaries, of course, will have to come out.

I am not upset about losing my ovaries. I am in menopause anyway.

The pelvic sonogram is scheduled for the next morning, a Friday. I am aware that a sonogram is routinely used with pregnant women to check the development of the fetus. But using it to find cancer is news to me.

The tech is a woman, in her early thirties, very gentle. "If you have any questions, just ask," she says. There is a computer screen beside her, to my right. The test is two-part, external and internal. The tech puts some gel on my stomach, then a card-shaped piece of equipment called a transducer near the left ovary. There are clumps of red dots on the screen that look like weather-radar pictures and seem to be moving.

I ask the tech what she's looking for. She explains: In order to grow, tumors often develop their own blood supply; she's checking for that now. She moves the transducer a few inches.

"Uh-huh, there it is," she says. "You can hear it."

She turns up the sound on the console. It's like hearing the ocean when you put your ear to a shell, but stronger. *Whoosh! Whoosh!* I know from women's movies on television that this is normally a big moment in sonography, the moment a woman hears her child's heartbeat for the first time, the heralding of a new life. It occurs to me now I may be hearing the opposite. What I am nurturing and carrying inside me may be my own death, or the beginnings of a death: a little death fetus.

The tech moves the transducer to the other side.

"Ahhh," she says, "There's one there, too."

By the time I've got my clothes on, I've diagnosed it ovarian cancer. I know just two things about ovarian cancer. It's vicious, and it killed Gilda Radner.

Surprise! I can't handle it. I go to my next appointment, my first in-person meeting with the shrink, as wired as if I've had ten cups of coffee. The doctor's name is David Payne, a bearded guy in his forties, with a nice roundness to him and an air of exceptional calm. The calm is probably a prerequisite for the job, I decide. They must test cancer shrinks for nerves, like police horses.

I'm afraid I have ovarian cancer, I tell Dr. Payne. That's what killed Gilda Radner. And she was more successful than me and she was funnier than me and she was married. If it's not ovarian cancer, it could be recurrent breast. Either way, I'm finished. And I'm afraid I'm gonna be finished fast. Like Debra Winger in *Terms of Endearment,* where she's lying exhausted in the hospital bed next to her tough little Shirley MacLaine mother, who's hollering at the nurses.

Payne doesn't bat an eye.

"That wasn't ovarian," Payne says. "It was another cancer." "Oh, yeah?" I say.

"Yeah," says Payne. "One of the doctors here was an adviser."

I'm impressed—this confirms the specialist mentality to which I am a slave. I settle in, and Dr. Payne tells me what I'm beginning to see is The Strategy: Do not make up frightening stories about the future. Stay with what you know. Gilda Radner is not you, everybody is different, and, also, Gilda Radner was sick years ago. There have been a lot of developments since then. If you find yourself morbidly obsessing about the future, distract yourself.

He also suggests drugs. I opt for a sedative called Klonopin, which he says is like Valium. I've put in a lot of air miles with Valium. I accept.

I am still scheduled to see my gynecologist, to redo the Pap smear. I also need to have my episode of irregular bleeding checked out with an endometrial biopsy. When Herb and I arrive at the office and tell the doctor what is happening, it seems to me I can actually see the color drain from the doctor's face.

Six weeks ago, the gynecologist said I was in great shape. Now, examining me, he tells me that the left ovary is slightly enlarged.

I have my first doubts about this man: Could the ovary have grown so quickly? Or did he miss something at the last visit? Still, I respect this doctor, and Norton likes him. If he has privileges at Memorial, I'll be happy to have him do the surgery. The doctor does not operate at Memorial. Not to worry, he says; he'll come visit me. But he never does. When the results of the Pap smear and the endometrial biopsy come in, they show everything to be normal.

IV

WITH MY FIRST CANCER, which I used to refer to as my big career break, when cancer was amusing, I had tried to protect my mother by stressing the good news: "It was malignant, but it's the best kind you can have, and they got it all out, so you don't have to come running up from Florida."

This time, though I still want to protect her, I am mature enough to accept that at 47 I still want my mother. It will also be a kindness to the people of Daytona Beach. My mother is wired. I picture her caroming through her morning walk around the mall, haranguing strangers with the details of medical reports.

"Money, thank God, is not an issue," she's probably saying right now to the checkout girl at the Winn Dixie.

She flies north, ready to pay whatever it takes to buy back my health.

"I got five big ones strapped to my you-know-what," she tells me from the airport.

"Drug dealers carry less cash than the people in your family," Herb says.

Then she and Herb and I go to Memorial to see the surgeon Norton has picked out for me.

His name is Richard Barakat, a good-looking, easygoing guy with a sweet, boyish style and a bit of a baby face. I make him to be maybe 38. Another middle-age milestone: My surgeon is younger than me. Women, I am sure, have always found him adorable. I see a line of aunts pinching his cheeks and hollering "Could you just eat him up?" for decades, maybe well into his thirties.

I like to tape important conversations with doctors, so I can listen to them as many times as I need and make sure I've got everything straight, but this seems to be against this department's policy. I figure it has to do with some recent bad press: A famous Indian actress brought her mother over for brain surgery, and they confused her with another Indian patient and operated on the wrong side of her head. Apparently, they're nervous.

Still, Barakat, after examining me, gives us the feeling that we can ask as many questions as we like. Herb and I take out our notebooks.

The ultrasound shows enlargement of both ovaries, with predominantly solid masses and neoplasms (new growths), Barakat says. After a woman's period stops, it is uncommon to get neoplastic cysts. The next issue is whether these new growths are malignant or benign. There are four things that can suggest malignancy: if the growths are bilateral; if the masses are solid; if there's increased blood flow; if there's fluid in the base of the pelvis. My ultrasound shows them all.

I am not panicked. From my conversations with the tech, this is what I expect. I can handle this.

"Four for four," I say.

Ma says nothing, which for her is unusual. She's just sitting there, rigid.

Herb tries to find us an out.

"Is there any chance this could still be benign?" he asks. There is a possibility, says Barakat. It happened recently with an elderly woman who had similar test results.

I'm thinking it is best to be realistic. "Did she have elevated blood markers?" I ask.

"No," Barakat says.

If, however, these masses are malignant and it's ovarian cancer, we're still catching the disease early, he says. Examining me, he felt no nodules at the base of the pelvis. The CAT scan shows no disease in the upper abdomen and no disease in the omentum. If it's malignant, the chances are three to one it will be ovarian cancer rather than metastatic breast cancer. The fact that the breast-cancer markers are up is not definitive—ovarian can also read on those blood tests. Bottom line: We'll know what I have only when the ovaries are removed.

The best way to remove the ovaries, Barakat says, is laparoscopy; it's "minimally invasive" surgery, in which four small incisions are made on the abdomen and they operate with the assistance of a tiny camera and a television monitor. The ovaries will be sent to the lab for a frozen-section diagnosis while I'm still on the table.

If the malignancy is metastatic breast cancer, there will be no further surgery. I'll be treated with chemotherapy, because the cancer is systemic— throughout my body.

If I have ovarian cancer, they'll do the larger surgery, removing the uterus, ovaries, and Fallopian tubes. They will also do a "staging" operation: take several biopsies from the abdomen to see whether the cancer has spread. Cancer is classified in stages from zero to four, determined by the size of the tumor or tumors and their distance from the origin. The earlier the stage, the better the prognosis. In the best scenario, all visible cancer can be removed at surgery.

I ask whether laparoscopy can be done with a local. Impossible, Barakat says.

He also confirms what I've suspected: A new primary cancer would be better than metastatic breast cancer.

"We've got very good treatment for ovarian," Barakat says. "The cure rate for first-stage ovarian cancer is 90 percent. Second-stage, it's 70 percent; third-stage—"

"Stop!!" I yell. We set surgery for eight days later, the Tuesday before Thanksgiving.

The shrink, Dr. Payne, has counseled distraction, so I try. I tell only a few close friends what's happening, because when I have to repeat the story, I get scared. I go to my friend Ben's 60th-birthday party, and when a Lifetime TV exec tells me they've bought my breast-cancer movie and that he hopes I'll be able to promote it, l lie.

"Absolutely!" I say.

I get the preop prep routine from Dr. Barakat's nurse, a motherly older lady with an Irish brogue who reminds me of the waitresses at Schrafft's who knew when to steer you away from the chicken salad. The one thing that bothers me is her habit of saying

"God forbid" whenever she says the word cancer. "The doctor will do a frozen section during the surgery, but we never go by that entirely; we go by the final pathology," she says when I ask her how soon I'll know what I've got. "If it is, God forbid, malignant, from what Dr. Barakat felt it looks fairly early. Nothing shows gross tumor, if, God forbid, it's ovarian cancer. Your abdomen is not all distended to your neck. I'll tell you one thing: Ovarian is very chemo-sensitive. Most patients respond very well. Unfortunately, they don't always stay in remission."

I have two sessions with Dr. Payne, who tells me he'll be in the recovery room when I wake up. Pretty neat, I think. An outside therapist could not do that.

Payne also encourages me to try to stop worrying about what will happen to me: When we have a diagnosis, I can think about it, he says, because then I'll be able to think constructively, to decide what I'm going to do.

He also asks me which cancer I am most afraid of.

I cannot say. I know a new primary is supposed to be better than recurrent cancer. But if it's ovarian, Larry Norton will not be my doctor: The breast-cancer department at Memorial has grown so large that he no longer heads both breast and ovarian medicine at Memorial, only breast. I've known Norton and my breast surgeon, Jeanne Petrek, for five years; they're my lifelines. I can't imagine fighting for my life with strangers.

My mother is staying with the family in the Catskills. Just like before, I ask her to wait and come in the day after surgery, so that, going in, I will not have to worry about her. I ask Don and my friend Heidi to join Herb at the hospital while I'm in surgery, so Herb will not be alone. Heidi has done this before for me, with the breast cancer. Don put in a month at St. Vincents when Rick was dying. It makes me sad. We are getting to be pros.

Surgery is scheduled for 7:30 in the morning. I'm told to get there an hour and a half early, like it's an international flight. Herb stays at my house the night before. He also honors Jewish time: We set two alarms. Neither goes off. At six, I wake up with a nightmare. I'm going somewhere important, and I'm missing the flight. I leap up, hollering to Herb.

"Think of it this way: They can't start without you," says Herb, throwing on his clothes.

"But they'll think I don't care," I say. "I don't care, they won't care. They'll do a quickie and go out for a nice breakfast. Or turn me over to the India brain man."

I had wanted a sedative, but there is no time. I'm with Herb only five minutes before they wheel me to preop, with its creepy dark lighting and the patients, on their gurneys, in a row, lying fiat and quiet as cadavers. Nurses are there, but they murmur, like they're getting you ready for the twilight zone of anesthetized sleep. The loneliest place in the world, I think.

Then there's Barakat, under the surgical lighting, looking fresh faced and gung ho and then—it seems no time at all has passed—there are faces and I'm awake. The faces appear at intervals: Herb's first, scared and worried; then, maybe, Dr. Payne, telling me I'm out of surgery and doing fine. There is a sharp line of pain running down my stomach: I feel as if I have been stabbed. I am happy to see Dr. Payne, I would like to talk to him, but it takes too much effort to get out the words. "Pain," I struggle to say and they give me more drugs.

Or maybe Dr. Barakat comes in before that.

"We tried to do the laparoscopy, but the disease had twisted around the bowel, so we had to do the bigger procedure," he is saying. "We got most of it out."

I am trying, through this haze of dope and pain, to form questions. Most of it?

"It was more advanced than we thought," Barakat says. "It had broken through the ovaries. There were spots on the omentum . . ." It seems to me he lists other places, that he speaks for some time. For me, it comes down to one thing: I have cancer all through me. I'm dead.

V

WHEN I WAS DIAGNOSED with breast cancer, the bad news was immediately coupled with the good: The lump in my breast was malignant, the surgeon told me twenty minutes after he'd removed it, but it looked like he'd gotten it all, and if that was true, the cure rate was very good—90 percent.

There were some moments of terror, some fear that cancer would show up in other parts of the body, but somehow, within minutes of getting the news, I had made an adjustment: "The position I'm taking is not that I have cancer, but that I had a cancer and they took it out," I told Herb. "Until it's proven otherwise, as far as I'm concerned that cancer is gone."

I was right—the cancer turned out to be a highly curable Stage Two.

With breast cancer, I felt more in control. The lump in my breast had been removed with a local, so

I was clearheaded. When it was out, I told the surgeon I wanted to see it. It was the size of a robin's egg and had been sliced down the middle. When the surgeon said the tumor seemed to be encapsulated, I could see that it was so.

And there was something else: The tumor—to me, the deceased tumor—was lying in a metal tray while I was up on my elbows sizing it up, so it seemed pretty clear who was in charge.

But this is different. I am not clearheaded when the surgeon talks to me; the drugs are pushing me down like a hand on my face. The cancer has not all been removed—it is worse than the sonogram indicated, and it has spread. I have had major surgery; the first few days, I am groggy with painkillers.

Memories are incomplete: My stomach, cut from my belly button to the top of my pubic hair and distended like one of the strange, football-shaped fruits at Balducci's. The wound closed with staples, like I am a Jiffy pack. Vaginal bleeding, frightening me, until somebody explains I've had a D&C and the bleeding is normal. A nurse replacing a sanitary napkin in front of Herb. Blood on the napkin. Looking at Herb and feeling terrible I am putting him through this. He isn't my husband; he didn't sign up for this.

We're the feature people. We do the jokes.

Learning from Herb that my mother, too anxious to stay away, had come to the hospital during surgery. But Herb thought that if I saw her unexpectedly, in the recovery room, I would be frightened, so Donal took her home. My beautiful, redheaded breast surgeon, Dr. Petrek, coming to visit.

"I talked to Larry Norton, and he says it's not as dire as it looks," she says.

"Dire?" He used the word *dire?* So why isn't it dire? But I don't remember the answer.

My mother, sitting in my room with the same expression she had when things had gotten bad with my father. An unending series of nurses and surgical residents and doctors, who put their stethoscopes to my stomach to listen for bowel sounds and try to determine whether my intestines have recovered from the trauma of surgery.

"Pass any gas?" they all ask.

The doctors still do not know if I have metastatic breast cancer or ovarian cancer. I also find, after our recovery-room chat, that I am afraid of Dr. Barakat. He stops outside my room, to brief the residents and fellows who follow him around the hospital and are even younger than he is, and when he does, I will myself not to hear. If he's telling them how much time I have left, I don't want to know.

When he comes in alone one day, Thanksgiving or the day before, I start to cry. I feel bad doing it, like I am letting down my side, though whether my side is writers or Wadlers I cannot say. "I just want to know if I have a shot," I say.

This is what I find interesting about surgeons: They can stand three hours with your intestines in their hands, but if you start to cry, they're lost.

"Don't cry," Barakat says—I think he says. "I've got my wife and kids waiting. How can I go home if you're crying?"

He says something reassuring about chemotherapy, what good medicine they have, but I do not recall being reassured. Then it's maybe six or seven in the evening, the senior staff seems to have gone home, and Norton walks into the room and sits down.

"Pass any gas?" he asks cheerfully. I have never been so happy to see him.

"It's Thanksgiving," I say. "Don't you have a home?"

And, after a bit, "Can you save me?"

He's in a philosophical mode, which happens with him sometimes.

"Can I save your life?" he says. "Well, you gotta be careful with hubris; finally, it's only God that can save lives, but yeah, yeah . . . I can save you."

Five days after surgery, they take the staples out of my belly and let me go home. The house is empty: Herb, who has been with me every day, is at his place. Mom is back in Florida; we both feel there is nothing much she can do. The wound at the base of my belly pulls when I walk as if it's going to rip. My intestines have gone on permanent strike.

I had not wanted people to know what was happening just yet, but I had not factored in Ma.

"She's in the hospital—oops, I wasn't supposed to tell you," she tells my friend Roberta when she calls, and that is that. The phone rings, the fax in my bedroom-office spits messages onto the floor that are supposed to be cheering: "A tragic illness is one in which someone does not lose any weight." What I feel, mostly, is a growing sense of distance. The world is divided into me and them, doomed and healthy, and only a few people, like Herb and Heidi and Ma, who were in the hospital with me, and Donal, who is under the shadow himself, can understand.

I pull out my medical-reference books and look up ovarian cancer, avoiding statistics on survival. They say the same thing: Ovarian cancer is asymptomatic in the early stages—One and Two. Because of this, it is usually not caught until it is advanced—Stages Three and Four. The prognosis then is "poor." I look at the publication dates to see whether the books are outdated. They are not so old as I would like.

A week after surgery, Norton phones.

"We got the reports," he says. "We're calling it ovarian." Calling it? It makes it sound like a disputed play in baseball.

No, says Norton, it's definitely ovarian, a Stage Three: Disease had spread out of the ovary, into the pelvis and abdomen, but it had not spread beyond the abdomen. He's seen the surgical report. The ovaries, Fallopian tubes, and omentum were removed. The D&C showed the uterus was clean; they left it in. Good news that it's a new primary and not a recurrence of breast cancer? He considers it great news. He outlines the battle plan: I'll have chemo; when it's over, they'll see if any cancer's left. God willing, there won't be.

"Y'know the reason we found this early has to do with my superb follow-up," he says, feeling relieved enough to joke. "I'm under a lot of pressure from people in my own community not to do those blood tests; it's considered excessive by modern standards."

"I don't know," I say. "Stage Three doesn't strike me as all that early."

"It's not extensive Stage Three," Norton says. "There wasn't a lot of disease in the abdomen. You didn't have bulky disease. What there was, was easily resected."

That is doctor talk, *resected;* it means "removed." Meanwhile, if things are so good, what about that conversation with Petrek, in which he allegedly used the word *dire?*

"Anytime a cancer is out of its place of origin, it's serious," he says. "Look, I'm not gonna bullshit you. We can't guarantee you a cure. But this is good."

What about Gilda Radner?

"I can never talk about another case," says Norton. "But her husband has written about it, and that cancer wasn't caught until very late. And they didn't have Taxol then. That's the big advance with the chemotherapy, Taxol."

"I'm glad it's settled," he says.

VI

IN FACT, THERE HAPPEN TO BE a lot of things that still are not settled for me. How long had the ovarian cancer been in me? Would sonograms have caught it earlier? If the uterus is routinely taken out for ovarian cancer, and what they saw in surgery might have been ovarian cancer, how come my uterus wasn't removed? Checking my medical records, I find a fourteen-month gap between visits to the gynecologist. Am I going to die because I was careless?

And then there is the big one: I am certain Larry Norton has saved my life, or at least extended it. But why, followed in the best cancer hospital in the country, did I have a cancer that wasn't spotted until it was a Stage Three?

Barakat, talking to me after the diagnosis, says with ovarian cancer they recommend a "second-look

47

surgery" when you've finished chemotherapy—and *then* they will take my uterus out.

This still doesn't make much sense to me: If you're in there—and it's not like going to the Korean market; one isn't in there that often—why not just remove the uterus? Nobody ever told me there could be a second surgery.

But I don't press. I have had a realization about cancer: You should not ask the question if you cannot handle the answer, and at the moment I can't. The treatment plan these guys are slowly unveiling to me is rough enough: "Second-look surgery." I'm going to have an operation like the one I just had *again?* I also don't think hearing negative survival odds are going to help. The numbers Barakat told me before surgery keep going through my head as it is: *First-stage ovarian cancer: 90 percent survival; second-stage, 70 percent.* Whatever the survival rate for Stage Three is, it can't be good. I throw out my medical books and ask two friends who do medical reporting to look into ovarian-cancer treatment for me and make sure Memorial is up to speed.

Then I call Ma.

"I'm thinking I'll get a little Miata, secondhand, and maybe you could help," I tell her.

"Secondhand?" she says. "Your father never bought a car secondhand. You know what your father said?" A pause, because my father is deceased, which in Judaism is all that is required to become a saint. "Your father said: 'Secondhand is trouble.'"

"Well, that will be a big change in my life," I say. "Secondhand. I'm not working. A convertible, red—"

"—Well, of course, red. What kind of a person would get a convertible that wasn't red?" Ma interrupts.

"—Decent sound system," I interrupt back. "Keep it to $10,000. Take one of your 5 million boyfriends to kick the tires or whatever guys do."

Ten days after surgery, when it still hurts if I climb stairs, Herb and I and our friend Max, who is one of my medical experts, go to meet my gynecological oncologist. His name is David Fennelly; he's Irish and slim, in his early thirties, and the minute I see him I know he is a good, ethical person. It's his eyes, I decide, trying to figure it out; he has extraordinarily kind eyes. He listens patiently while I talk about my history. When he speaks, it's with a brogue.

"Ovary cancer," he calls what I have. No, he says, he does not believe my doctors and I missed anything. The spotting I had is not something normally associated with ovary cancer. The *usual* presentation with ovary cancer is abdominal distension and a change in bowel habits, either constipation or diarrhea. That makes diagnosis tricky; people often have trouble with their bowels.

"That really gets to one of the problems we have with ovary cancer," he says. "It doesn't give us any clues at an early stage . . . but what you should know is we do have very effective treatment for you. In terms of prognosis for this type of disease, you're in a situation that is optimum."

Herb and Max and I are stunned.

"Optimum?" I say.

"Optimum in terms of your likely results and successes with chemotherapy," he says.

I can't believe it.

"Even with Stage Three?" I ask.

"What I say to patients who present with ovary cancer . . . the factors I'm concerned about are obviously the extent of the disease, but more importantly the amount of disease that's left after surgery," Fennelly says. "That's the most predictive factor. You really didn't have any disease left at the end of surgery. You've been what we call *optimally debulked.*"

This is a new and fabulous phrase. There are three writers in the room; we sit there enthralled and delighted with it, as if we've been shown a new toy. Max and Herb want to start playing with it right away.

"We considered Joycie optimally debulked all along," says Max.

I'm still having trouble absorbing the information.

"I was told, after surgery, that cancer had been left," I say.

"Optimally debulked means the vast majority of the disease is gone," says Fennelly. "We don't assume that we got everything out, or you wouldn't need chemotherapy. But the best group to be in is that group of patients that have had the majority of their disease resected. That gives chemotherapy the maximum chance to be effective. It's your type of patients who are cured."

We talk a good hour after that: My chemotherapy, Fennelly says, will be Cisplatin, a drug that's been used for a long time with ovarian cancer, and Taxol, the drug Norton had mentioned, and which I now think of as Taxol the Wonder Drug. Taxol the Wonder Drug is given in a 24-hour infusion and requires an overnight stay in the hospital;

Cisplatin, also given intravenously, takes an hour. For my first chemo, they will keep me in the hospital two days. They'll monitor my response to the drugs by giving me a special blood test for ovarian cancer, CA-125. CA-125 has not proved very effective in catching early disease, Fennelly says. It's neither sensitive enough nor specific enough, but it works very well for this. The major side effects of Cisplatin are nausea and vomiting, but we have medications that can control that pretty well these days. Cisplatin may also affect my sense of taste and cause neuropathy—numbness—in my fingers and toes. Taxol the Wonder Drug, in ten days to a week, will make me lose my hair. It has also been known to trigger allergic reactions, including a drop in blood pressure, facial flushing, and rapid heartbeat. To counteract that, I'll be given steroids. Steroids also help combat nausea.

I took a small amount of steroids with the chemotherapy I had for breast cancer. They left me wired and tearful and combative and ravenous. Now I don't care. I don't care that the neuropathy could make it difficult to write; I don't care that I'm going to lose my hair.

Herb and Max and I are so happy; we leave the office floating.

"For the first time, I think I could beat this," I say. "I feel like this is the first good news we've got."

"Me too," says Herb.

VII

ONE TIME, AT A PARTY, a woman who is the daughter of concentration-camp survivors tells the Middle-aged Mutant Jewish Writer a story: Her mother, who was Polish, had been stunningly beautiful, the woman says. She was also well educated. She had been taken to a concentration camp; her head had been shaved. Toward the end of the war, realizing that they were losing, the Germans took a group of Jewish prisoners, including the woman, out on a ship and pushed them overboard. The woman had seen her parents murdered; her sister's newborn child had been thrown by the Nazis from a hospital balcony. She did not resist when the officer came toward her. "Do what you will, I no longer care," she said, in German. Her German was perfect; her hair had grown back. The officer suddenly saw the woman not as a subhuman prisoner

55

but as a fellow human being. He threw a canvas sheet over her, and the woman lived.

I once spent six months in a country where I could not speak the language; hearing this story, I focused on the part about being able to speak. It is true, I think, that if someone is unable to speak your language, you dismiss her. But now, knowing that I will be bald in two weeks, I focus on the part of the story about hair. I will never let a doctor or nurse see me bald, I decide. I will never make it easy to separate me from them. Herb and I go to a wig store. Herb, who hates to shop, is suddenly very interested: He wants me to try on a long blonde *Baywatch* number.

"Oh, Herb, not you, too?" I say.

He grins, the way he did when we were in Paris and he saw his first topless television commercial.

"Just once," he says. "For me."

I do it, but I realize, somewhat to my surprise, that what I want now is to look like myself: I choose a reddish brown, my own unnatural color.

Then I get ready for the hospital. A year earlier, at the Dana Farber Cancer Institute in Boston, a Boston *Globe* medical writer with breast cancer died from an overdose of chemotherapy. If a medical writer isn't safe in a hospital, I think, what could they do to a feature person like me? I make a deal with Herb: We'll carry notebooks, we'll learn what my dosage should be, we'll check it. I pack tights and Hawaiian shirts, so I won't look like a sick person, and old rock-and-roll and show tunes.

Chemotherapy begins in early December, two weeks after surgery. The drugs start before I even get to the hospital: Twenty milligrams of Decadron, a steroid, the night before to prevent that allergic reaction to Taxol the Wonder Drug; another twenty milligrams in the morning. At the hospital, the chemo is delayed four hours. I get an extra twenty milligrams of steroids and meet the parade of caretakers.

When the chemo nurse finally arrives, Herb and I check out the plastic bag with my name on it. My dose is supposed to be 175 milligrams per meter squared; it's given according to body weight, which comes to 297.5 milligrams. I ask the nurse to hoist it, to make sure it feels right, which was how El Al security once found a bomb in a piece of luggage in a story I covered. Then the nurse finds a vein in my arm for the IV drip.

I'm tense—Fennelly has said if there is an allergic reaction it happens right away. But I'm not tense long: the nurse starts the drip with cimetidine and Benadryl, to counteract the symptoms. The Benadryl makes me sleepy. In about fifteen minutes, the nurse starts the Taxol. No problem. Herb hangs around for a half-hour to make sure things are all right.

"Say good night, Gracie," he says, which is what he says when I've had a glass of wine and get sleepy. Then he goes home.

I wake up at seven that evening, famished and raring to go. The IV is hooked up to a hospital pole, so I can travel. I go down to the cafeteria, then decide to cruise the dayroom. I could get lucky, find a guy with something minor, a skin cancer, maybe.

I haul the pole, which has become my new best friend, to the dayroom. No one is there but a white-haired woman in a bathrobe who wants to know if I'm here for bingo and a group of Junior League types, stuffing Christmas baskets. They're all in bright Ladies Who Lunch suits and they're all blonde, except for one plump brunette, who I assume is their token. I look at them, and I am enraged. Is this conspicuous charity supposed to make anybody feel better but themselves? And the question that really bothers me: Why are they healthy when I'm not? A year from now, I will look at this and know it is steroids working, or at least partly steroids; now all I feel is rage. I step into the library to see if they have any of my stuff. They don't. Now I'm really peeved.

The next morning, I become aware of a roommate on the other side of the curtains. She's perhaps 70, with patchy short gray hair and a heavy Spanish accent. She is very sick. She throws up every twenty minutes, and usually, instead of ringing for a nurse, she gets up and carries her pail of vomit to the bathroom. Dr. Fennelly is also her doctor. I overhear parts of their conversation. My roommate is vomiting because she has tumors in her stomach. I am getting frightened: The woman in the bed across from me has ovarian cancer, and she is dying. Not today, not this week. But she is terminally sick with my cancer.

I wait for the woman to go to the bathroom, then I call Fennelly's office for reassurance.

The nurse is kind.

"That's the problem with being in the hospital— you see some of the sickest people," she says. "If you were to come to the clinic and see some of the outpatients, you'd see people who are doing very well ... most everyone responds to these drugs." If my roommate is really disturbing me, the nurse adds, I can ask whether another room is available.

I decide against changing rooms. Any harm to me has already been done. And if I leave, my roommate might realize it's because I think she's dying and don't want to be around her. I might make her feel worse.

I get my Walkman, put on *Guys and Dolls*, and try to separate and remember the good things about my case, the way Dr. Payne has taught me: "My doctor has told me I am in a good prognostic group. I have a good chance of a cure. Every body is different."

It doesn't work. On the tape, a make-believe gambler is singing that when you see a guy reach for stars in the sky, you can bet that he's doing it for some doll. Beyond that, the woman in the next bed is throwing up. I get up and go to my bag and find some almond skin cream that I've swiped from a hotel and a pair of pink socks and go visit. I find when I'm tired, a foot massage helps, I tell my roommate. I rub her feet, and she tells me her story:

She had had breast cancer, and then, years later, she got ovarian cancer and she went to a hospital on Long Island where they told her she had six months to live. She had never been followed with blood tests. A doctor she used to baby-sit for got her to Memorial. That was two years ago. She has three tumors in her stomach, and they're discussing surgery to put in a shunt so she can get rid of the fluids. She is tired of chemo and surgery, but she has grandchildren. She does not want her grandchildren to think she did not do everything she could to stay with them. Also, it turns out, she is not 70—she is 50. She was diagnosed with ovarian cancer at my age.

I go back to my side of the room. At midnight, I wake up, sweating. An unwelcome thought has muscled its way to the surface. The nurse has said most everyone responds to this chemotherapy, but if that is true, why is ovarian cancer such a deadly disease? It must be recurrence—the drugs work for a short time, then the cancer comes back. And what if I don't even reach that point? What if these drugs never work for me? I want to call Herb, but that's out. I can't say, "I'm scared, they gave me a roommate who's dying"; my neighbor might hear me.

I get up and take a walk around the floor. The corridors are empty. Why aren't the goddamn chaplains and shrinks and volunteers here at midnight, I think, when it's loneliest and most frightening? Whose bright idea was it to put somebody who's having her first chemo in with somebody who's dying? Why can't it be like college— freshmen room with freshmen?

I find a young nurse at the nursing station. The steroids are probably contributing to this, I say, embarrassed at being such a baby, but I'm really scared. I look at my roommate, who is dying, and I'm afraid I'm looking at my future.

The nurse is not sympathetic.

"How do you know she's dying?" she says accusingly.

"We're in the same room," I say. "There's a curtain between us. You hear everything. She may not be dying now, but she is dying. You can't help but know it."

The nurse's tone is recriminating.

"That's not true," the nurse says. "I saw you earlier: You were in there talking to her."

Herb and Donal take me home the next morning. I have no nausea. The pills I go home with, Kytril and Decadron—still more steroids—take care of that. I take them for five days. They are so strong that most of the time, I sleep. But it is not a good sleep. It's laced with nightmares, and even when I'm up, things feel unreal. I am jumpy and anxious.

The physical side effects of the Taxol and Cisplatin kick in: My appetite disappears. My mouth and tongue are coated. Coffee and orange juice have a strange metallic taste. The weekend after chemo, in an attempt at normalcy, I tell Herb I'd like to go to a movie. I choose a Western, because there is no cancer in Westerns. The movie opens with the hero's coffin being lowered into the ground. I start crying. *That's going to be me*, I think. The next day, there is a feature in the Sunday Times about a woman dying of ovarian cancer. Just like my roommate, she was diagnosed two years ago.

I put in a call to Payne. He thinks I'm having a reaction to the steroids. He suggests an increase in sedatives as well as a mental counterattack. "Tell yourself, when you get scared, 'This will pass. This is drugs.'"

Eight days after chemo, I can taste again—the orange juice I have in the morning is the best juice I've ever had. I'm done with the anti-nausea drugs; I'm no longer wired.

I find the card of a patient representative I met in the hospital and call her up and talk to her about the nurse.

A person without compassion has no place in a cancer hospital, I say. I am weak when I am in the hospital and I cannot protect myself, but I am not weak now. I have five more chemotherapy sessions. I never want to see that nurse in my room again.

VIII

My hair starts falling out ten days after chemotherapy: a few strands on a white tablecloth at the Knickerbocker restaurant. I am having lunch with a guy I met at a party two months ago. The guy is sniffly. "I'm fighting something off," he says. "Me too," I say.

I wait a few days, till my hair comes out in clumps in the shower, then, as directed, I go back to Bitz 'N Pieces, a wig store on the West Side, where they shave the rest of my hair and do the final fit for the wig. They don't like to buzz you until the hair is really coming out. They say it's too traumatic.

"Why didn't you tell me? I would have gone with you," Heidi says afterward. And, "Did you cry?"

I didn't cry because I was steeled for it. Also because when I spoke to women about breast cancer, a lot of them told me they'd lost their hair and it was no big deal. It grew back; they had gotten a chance to play around with all these nifty wigs.

I can handle this, I think when they take me into a private little room.

One wall is mirrored. As the hair comes off, I decide I look like a recruit going into basic training. When I get home, I take off my wig and all my clothes, and stand in front of a full-length mirror and check me out naked. I am quite astonishingly bald, but I am still dramatically girly: My waist goes in, almost everything else goes out. I look sort of sci-fi. On the Starship *Enterprise,* they would probably go for me in a big way. Space Tomato, I call me. Maybe I should take out a personals ad: Mature Woman seeks Trekkie.

The bald aspect can be dealt with. It's the dead aspect that's giving me trouble. Going to renew my driver's license, I see that my new one will expire in five years and I have a disturbing thought: Who is going to expire first, me or my license?

IX

FENNELLY HAS AN EXTRAORDINARILY soothing style. If the theater were on fire—which, it occurs to me, my theater is—this is the guy you'd want to make the announcement. But the more we talk, the more of a wild ride I see this cancer is going to be. In a meeting with Fennelly, to adjust my anti-nausea drugs, he has given me the results of my first ovarian blood screen: 860. Normal is between 1 and 35. If the number isn't significantly down after the third treatment, Fennelly says, he'd be "concerned." I mentally translate from the Fennelly to the Wadler: *Concerned*—what you'll be doing New Year's Eve in the year 2000 is no longer a problem.

The CA-125 blood test, Fennelly continues, is done every third week when I come to the hospital for chemo. I can call for the results five days later. A nurse clarifies the drill: I'll get my test results from a nurse. Unless the numbers are up. Then I'll have to wait and speak to the doctor. I get tense just thinking about it: You make a call and find out if you're going to live or die. If your doctor phones just to see how you're doing, and leaves his name on your machine, you'd probably die of stroke.

I call up Donal, who has been living with the knowledge that he is HIV-positive for three years, and ask him how he manages to deal with this level of life-and-death uncertainty.

"Well, think about it," he says. "I've always been good at repression."

"I'm supposed to be learning that, sort of," I say. "Distraction."

"You're not so good," Donal says.

This is true. What I need now, I decide, is a success story. I call Share, a support-and-information group for women with breast and ovarian cancer, and tell them I'd like to talk to a woman who had Stage Three ovarian cancer and is at least five years out. Two days later, a woman calls. She had a tumor the size of a grapefruit pressed up against her liver. She had been treated, pre—Taxol the Wonder Drug, with Cytoxan and Cisplatin. This was six years ago. She's fine. In fact, though she knew she had a cancer that could kill her she had known from the beginning she would be fine.

"That's what I'm having trouble with, getting my confidence back," I tell her. "With the first cancer, I did really well. Really." Like maybe she won't believe me. "And now I just can't seem to get back on the horse, or whatever the expression is."

"That's like comparing the book and the movie," she says. "They're two different things. What's to be gained by comparing?"

I cobble together a chemotherapy plan with Payne: He suggests a private room. It will cost $165 more. For protecting myself, it's worth it.

Herb and I have not been romantic since I was 29. We are best friends, but in certain areas, Herb likes to maintain a distance. I have never met his mother, for example, because Herb believes that if we met, one or both of us would complain about the other until one or both of us were dead, and he could not take it. When we were dating, if I left a pair of socks at his place, he got tense.

Now this changes.

For chemo two, in mid-December, I check into my private room, and I do not leave it. For the next week, until the drugs are out of my system, Herb lives with me in my apartment. He sleeps on the living-room couch; and in the morning we switch rooms and Herb moves into my bedroom-office and writes.

Sometimes, when we wake up, I get into the big queen-size sofa bed with Herb and we have coffee and read the papers together. If I am too tired to read, Herb reads the funniest stuff out loud. It's a terrible winter, a winter of record-breaking storms, but inside, making fun of the news together, we are snug.

"Is it the drugs, or have we mellowed?" I ask him.

"Drugs," Herb says. "Tomorrow you won't remember any of this."

In the evenings, however, the terrors still get me. Around 6:30, for the first five nights after chemo, when the steroids are in me, I cry. Sometimes I cry on the phone to my mother in Florida; sometimes I cry to Herb: I'm dying, I say. I've had two cancers; who ever beats two cancers? Why me? I didn't hurt anybody. Okay, maybe I wrote some snotty stories about movie stars, but I can't see this pissing off God, unless it's actors who are the chosen people. Which is really depressing.

Herb doesn't know what to do. He calls me Joycel, a variation on Joycela, my Yiddish name, which only people who know me very well and like me call me.

"You're not gonna die, Joycel," he says. "I'm not gonna let you die." For years, whenever we meet each other and leave each other, we quack; I am not certain why. When we are very relieved to see one another, we quack a lot. Herb takes a shot.

"C'mon, Joycel, give me a quack," he says.

"Aaaaaghh," I say, crying.

"That's not such a great quack," he says.

"Aaaagggg?" I say. "Ack?"

Then something hits me.

"You remember that part in *Garp*," I say, "where the gunner who got shot can only say his name—Garp—and then he gets worse and he can't remember the *G* and he can only say 'Arp,' and then he loses the *p*? That's what's happening to me."

And we're laughing and I feel better.

X

WHEN MUTANT JEWISH WRITER had breast
cancer, the chemotherapy she was given was
"prophylactic"—a preventative to try to keep any
unseen cancer cells from coming back. With ovarian
cancer, it's very different: The doctors know there is
cancer left in me after surgery. I also know that if I
don't respond to chemotherapy, that's bad.

"This is your best shot, right?" I say to my
gynecological oncologist, David Fennelly, during my
first treatment with Taxol and Cisplatin. "So, what if
these drugs don't work?"

"We could have a very depressing conversation
about that," Fennelly says, "but as a medical doctor,
I'd rather not." He also warns me that the results of
my first CA-125 blood screens, the test for the
presence of ovarian cancer cells, might not be an
accurate reflection of how well the chemotherapy is
working—my recent surgery could throw it off. I don't

call the doctor's office, then, for the test results of my first chemo. Why drive myself crazy?

Soon after the numbers are in, however, I need to talk about something else with Larry Norton, my breast-cancer oncologist at Memorial Sloan-Kettering.

"Congratulations. I saw your test results. You're doing great!" he says as soon as he picks up the phone.

He punches up my records on the computer. My CA-125, at the start of chemotherapy, had been 860; after one hit, it's 690. I call Herb, then my mother.

"You know," Ma says, "it wouldn't hurt you to go to a synagogue this Friday and thank You-Know-Who."

"Why?" I say. "For giving me two You-Know-Whats?"

"For giving the doctors the brains to find it early," Ma says.

"Actually, a Stage Three cancer is not so early," I say.

"Yes it is," says Ma.

The next day I get a call from my old boyfriend Donal. He's been HIV-positive for more than two years, and his health the past few months has been worrisome. The T-cell count for a healthy person is

1,200. Donal's count is under 400. In the past month, however, he's heard news of a new treatment, at an outfit called the Aaron Diamond Research Center. He's just had his first interview there. It's unlike anything he's ever heard of; it will involve three drugs, one a protease inhibitor. His voice breaks and he starts to cry. I am frightened. Donal never cries.

"Is something wrong?" I say. "Did they find something?"

"No," says Donal. "It's just I've held it in so long—and now, if what they told me is right, for the first time there's hope. Who knows? Maybe we'll both beat it."

So we go on. I had figured, with chemo once every three weeks, I could still have a normal life: I might be knocked out one week, but in the remaining two I would make up for it. I could also work.

"Cancer is perfect for television," I tell my friend Sybil, who is a comedy writer. "You pitch, you get sick, it takes them three weeks to get back to you, by that time you're up again." "I can see you're new to this business," Sybil says. "Actually, you could die, have an out-of-body experience, come back, and you'd still be waiting for them to get back to you."

But things don't work out that way.

I grow more tired after each chemo, sleeping ten days, then twelve. I cannot concentrate enough to write. When I can taste food, the steroids make me ravenous: I gain fifteen pounds. Bald, which I originally thought I could handle, is difficult. I am trying to be game—I have four wigs now, including two blonde ones—but they can't hide everything. I am puffy and moon-faced from steroids; my eyebrows are gone; I'm down to six or seven eyelashes. When I wake up in the morning, before I've painted on eyebrows and cheekbones and faked lashes with eyeliner, my face has the contours of a bowling ball. Surgery has marked me. The scar bisecting my belly now puckers in. The more weight I gain, the deeper the indentation.

There's a nude photo of me on my bedroom wall Donal took when we first started going out—that's how you know a photographer is in love, with you or with somebody else; he takes pictures. I'm standing in front of a vanity in a hotel bathroom with one hand behind my head, doing a spoof on a pin-up pose. My hair is shoulder-length. I curve like a Varga girl. The bathroom is mirrored, so the image is doubled: two Varga girls. I am 32 years old, the New York correspondent for the Washington *Post*. I have a

---

boyfriend who chases me around the house with a hard-on.

I look at the picture a lot: I had so much hair. My stomach was so smooth. I was so healthy.

The chemotherapy keeps working. After my second treatment, the CA-125 drops from 690 to 245; after the third, it's down to 63; after the fourth, it's 33—I hit normal.

Donal, who is being treated across the street from Memorial, at Rockefeller University, on the new protease cocktail, is having even more dramatic results: In one month, his viral load goes from 100,000 to undetectable. We have a celebration dinner with Herb and some old friends from Budapest, and Donal takes out his mahogany pillbox and spreads the pills he has to take three times a day on the table. We look at them, the little pills that are saving his life—the combination, had it been discovered two years earlier, that might have saved his boyfriend. Three writers are at the table, and this time, words fail.

But I still can't shake the fear.

I have my sports car now. It's a little red Miata; one of the widowers in love with my mother found it. It is perfect, it is the car of my dreams, but I have nightmares about it: My little red car is stolen. My little red car is wrecked. I am dead and my mother and her friend are in my car driving fast on the beach, like Shirley MacLaine and Jack Nicholson in *Terms of Endearment*. My mother gets to live because she is better at life than I am. She does not brood and worry. She would not carry a torch for some guy for four years. She manages to find boyfriends.

I talk about it with David Payne, my psychologist at the hospital. This is a curable cancer, he tells me; why not believe I will be among the people who will be cured?

I've had two cancers, I tell him. I can't believe I'm terrifically lucky.

He tries another tack, what I've come to think of as the Live-in-the-Moment Number.

"We don't know the future," he says. "Why fantasize about it? Do you feel better when you worry? Distract yourself."

I'm with him in concept. But I still can't stop worrying and asking questions.

Straightening out a problem with Blue Cross, I order a copy of my surgical report.

"Tell me you didn't read it," Herb says.

"Of course I read it," I tell him, dragging it out. "Listen to this: 'Adhesions of the sigmoid to the left side of the uterus.' I thought the uterus was clean.

You think that caused the constipation?" Herb is turning green.

"This is starting to feel like *Manhattan Murder Mystery,* the gastrointestinal version," he says.

In March, after four and a half months, I'm done with chemotherapy.

Second-look surgery, which is performed in ovarian cancer to see if any cancer is left after chemotherapy, is questioned by some doctors. They believe it's unnecessary trauma, and if the cancer comes back, you'll eventually see it in elevated blood markers.

But it seems logical to me. The only way the doctors know for certain how effective the chemo has been is to see it under the microscope, and if I have any cancer left, I want to attack it early. Though my CA-125 blood tests, after the last three hits of chemotherapy, have been under 35—the cutoff for a normal reading—they've been only just normal: 33, 27, 34. I have a suspicion some microscopic cancer cells are still there.

Even if the cancer is gone, the doctors favor additional chemotherapy. According to my surgeon Dr. Richard Barakat, more than 50 percent of ovarian-cancer patients who seem to be cancer-free at second-look surgery recur in two years.

Interperitoneal therapy—chemo delivered to the abdomen—delays recurrence and may even prevent it. The drugs are administered through a medical port implanted just below the ribs during second-look surgery. I hate surgery, but I like the idea of interperitoneal: If I could remove my abdominal cavity and soak it overnight in the sink with chemo, I would. There is also that pesky uterus to get out.

Why wasn't the uterus taken out the first time?

People tend to think you can just pop organs out, "like a chip shot," Barakat tells me and Herb. It's not always like that.

Herb and I would never set foot on a golf course, but we get the picture.

The uterus was, um, stuck?

There was a sheeting of cancer between the rectum and the uterus, Barakat says. To remove the uterus at first surgery, he would have had to "resect"—remove—a section of the colon. They do a fair amount of colon surgery with ovarian patients, so they "probably" would have been able to put it together again—*oy, probably?* But two things made him decide against it.

If I had metastatic breast cancer, treatment would not necessitate removing the uterus. In that case, the cancer would be systemic and best treated with chemotherapy; it would have been wrong to risk the complications of bowel surgery to remove a little bit of cancerous plaque. If I had ovarian cancer, the plaque would probably be dissolved by chemotherapy and the uterus could be easily removed at second look. I'm beginning to see why the surgical puppies follow him so closely.

And no, by the way, when he did my first surgery, he did not see any mass that could cause constipation.

We set the date for surgery, and Barakat and I make a deal: No matter what he sees, good news or bad, no matter how much I pump him, as, he insists, I did last time, he will not tell me what he finds until I am recovered from anesthesia.

It's April. I have a seven-week vacation between chemo and surgery. I pick up my car in the mountains and take it back to the city, following 9W along the Hudson and down the mountain on the Storm King Highway, a drive that does for me what going to the synagogue does for my mother. I get a press-on tattoo for my fuzzy but still primarily bald head, for surgery. (LUCKY, with two dice, is the one I wanted, but the store is out.)

The recovery-room experience this time seems cloudy and pink, but that is probably projection: I open my eyes and there is Barakat's face, happy and extraordinarily boyish in his blue-green surgical cap. "I didn't see anything," he says. (I think he says.) "We still have to wait for the lab results, but it looks clean. I know I wasn't supposed to tell you, but I thought you'd want to know. That's okay right?"

I float away in my blue paper surgical hats much easier the second time around. Wonder if they changed the drugs? Herb materializes with Ma. Seems to be waiting for something. "Don't you have something to show your mother?" Herb says. Oh, right: Cue the actor. I manage to push my cap back, to show Ma the tattoo on the left side of my head, where you'd wear a beret. It has a red rose. MOTHER, it says.

The biopsy results take three days.

"Before you tell me anything, I just want to know, even if you found something, that there's something you can do," I tell Barakat when he walks in, trailing residents.

He looks serious.

"There was something," Barakat says. "We did 25 biopsies. We found microscopic cells in two of them, in the colon and in the uterus. There was no lymph-node involvement. We also found some cells in an abdominal wash."

I'm disappointed, but I'm not surprised or terrified. My CA-125 test had been barely normal. I can handle this. "That still seems pretty good," I said.

Barakat agrees.

"It is," he says. "There's one study that patients with microscopic disease at second look do as well as patients with no disease, when treated with peritoneal. We can cure you. In fact, I'll tell you something else."

I'd rather this act end on the good news.

"Don't tell me," I say.

"No," he says, "let me tell you: There's another study that says you are in a population 50 percent of whom survive at least four years."

I'm stunned.

"You consider this good news?" I say.

But he has wanted so to tell me, I know that to him, it is.

XI

THE MUTANT HAS THREE or four of Larry Norton's 5 billion phone numbers, but she tries to save her calls for emergencies. Pull Norton out of the lab at the wrong minute, she figures, it could take five years longer for the cure for cancer. Also, he had a habit, when she called him once or twice during chemotherapy, of asking how the work was going or telling her inspirational stories about ballplayers.

"Doing any writing?" he'd ask. "You know, a lot of my patients do their best work in this period."

"Work?" I would say, astonished. "I'm having trouble walking down the street."

Being told that I have a 50 percent chance of surviving four years, however, qualifies as an emergency, so I call Norton at home. He's traveling. A few hours later, the phone rings and Norton materializes in an airport in Atlanta:

Shazam! My own fairy godperson! I had always hoped for one, though I'd never figured the area of specialization would be cancer. Though maybe that's what a fairy godperson is when you are middle-aged: the doctor who is head of the department.

I hit Norton with the 50 percent statistic, expecting he'll do what he always does: make a joke about surgeons or tell me about a new treatment in the works.

Only this time, he doesn't.

"Fifty percent is 50 percent," he says. "It's still a shot." That's the best he can offer, a shot?

"You gotta think positive," Norton says. "Let me tell you a story about a ballplayer I once treated."

"I know this story," I tell him.

"There was this baseball player I treated, very famous—you know I can't reveal names," Norton says. "I asked him why he hit so many home runs and he said he just knew he would, and if he happened to strike out, he just sat down on the bench, knowing next time he was up at bat, he would hit a home run. Which he did. He had this irrational optimism, which is why he was so successful—"

"No, no, this gets into making the patient responsible for everything; it's a terrible metaphor," I say.

"It's a great story," Norton says. "Actually, I do think the way you think about things matters. But that's not the point. The point is, you have to get up there every time like you're going to win. You have to do that for your life. It's how you look at a thing, like is the glass half full or half empty . . ."

"But *I'm* the glass, see?" I tell Norton.

"You can't be one of those people who become obsessed with their disease," Norton says. "That happens, the cancer wins. What you have to do is concentrate on living."

I get off the phone feeling gloomy. I've felt safe with Norton on my side, but if he was as powerful as I like to think, we'd be praying in Temple Norton.

"What do you want the doctors to tell you?" Payne asks the next time we speak.

"I want them to guarantee that I'm going to live," I say. "And they can't."

XII

IN THE INTEREST OF SCIENCE or the interest of the Mutant but not, she suspects, in the interests of both—the gynecological-service doctors, after second-look surgery, offer the Mutant a choice of treatment. She may have weekly Taxol for fifteen weeks, with a belly wash of Cisplatin every three weeks, or she may opt for a new, phase-one trial involving high-dose chemotherapy that probably won't be fatal.

The doctor making the offer is not David Fennelly, who is returning to Ireland, but the Mutant's new gynecological oncologist. Herb and Ma and I go in to see him two weeks after second-look surgery, in late May. The description he gives us of the high-dose treatment is grim:

Stem cells, young blood vessels that can multiply and grow to produce mature blood cells, would be "harvested" from my bloodstream in three or four painless, outpatient procedures. Then I would be given one high-dose treatment of Taxol, followed by two high-dose treatments of the drugs Thiotepa and Mitoxantrone. The theory is that the big blasts of chemo could finish off the resistant cancer cells for good. The "toxicity," however, would be major. Blood counts would drop severely. Three days after each treatment, I would need to be "rescued" with my own blood cells.

"For a short while, you'd be sicker than you ever have been in your life," says the doctor. "You'd have a raw gut; sometimes there are mouth sores so that you can't eat or drink. There's diarrhea, abdominal pain. It's potentially toxic to the heart . . ."

I feel a little ill.

"My heart? That's one of my favorite parts," I say weakly, and I am not joking.

The results of the new treatment?

It's too early to say. They've only treated four ovarian patients with this particular high dose. One, who like me had microscopic cancer at second look, is fine one year later; one has just entered the trial; two, with very-late-stage cancer, have recurred.

What does the doctor recommend?

"I don't push one or the other," he says. "It comes down to whether you're the kind of person who likes to go with a tried-and-true or you want to take a risk for a potential benefit that's unknown. It's a reasonable risk; they're both very good treatments. There are two things that shouldn't influence you: You're at very low risk of dying from the treatment and for getting leukemia."

There's something a little offensive to me here: a suggestion of something having to do with character, which is almost a challenge. I do not feel a life-or-death decision should come down to the "kind of person" I am. It should be based on the kind of treatment the hospital has to offer.

The doctor adds a frightening footnote, upping the ante:

If the cancer comes back after the treatment I choose, they will not be able to cure me. They will be able to treat me, and perhaps beat the cancer back for a time, but will not, with the current available drugs, cure me.

The doctor gives us all copies of the seven-page "Informed Consent for Clinical Research," which describes the trial, to take home. It's even more frightening than his description. "Ovarian cancer that has spread beyond the ovary and into the pelvis and abdomen and that persists following initial chemotherapy is usually not curable," it begins, a surprise to me, because from my discussion with Barakat, I'd gathered it often could be cured.

"Unanticipated side effects may occur...," it continues, which I figure is their legal catchall.

"... Fatal side effects may occur."

Nope. That's the catchall.

The effects of high-dose cyclophosphamide, high-dose Thiotepa, and high-dose Mitoxantrone take three paragraphs to list: They include risk of infection; bleeding; nausea; vomiting; loss of hair; sore mouth; loss of taste; watery diarrhea; heart, liver, skin, brain, lung, bladder damage. Kidney damage is possible but "uncommon." "Body fluid and electrolyte abnormalities may occur, and these may lead to seizure."

Ma is so scared she asks if I have any wine in the house, a request she usually makes only on Passover.

I don't know what to do.

The old Special Forces Wadler in me, which I fear has been triggered by my conversation with my new doctor, feels that if there is a stronger treatment, I've got to have it:

"Are you a sissy?"

"Sir, no, sir! Private Wadler is not a sissy, sir! I must add, sir, my being here is a major mistake and somebody is gonna hang. See, *I know the head of the department!*"

On the other hand, I have no evidence that the stronger drugs will work better.

When I call my new oncologist back, to press him for the hard figures I need to make a decision, he makes "an educated guess" that perhaps 60 to 70 percent of patients in my condition, treated with Taxol and interperitoneal therapy, will be alive at five years—not disease-free, he cautions, *alive*. Compared with the 50 percent recurrence rate of a dangerous trial, that looks pretty good to me.

I am frightened of what I'll find when I start reporting, but it's time. Heidi searches the online news services; Cheryl and Sybil and I read medical abstracts from the National Institute of Health and Oncolink.

The best news is not good: Taxol the Wonder Drug, used in combination with Cisplatin, does extend the life of women with advanced ovarian cancer by 50 percent. In real time, it's not such a fabulous feat. With the older combination, Cisplatin and cyclophosphamide, patients with ovarian cancer had a median survival of 24 months. Taxol used with Cisplatin raised the median survival to just 37 months. Resistance to chemotherapy and recurrence are common. There are high-dose trials all over the country.

I need second opinions. Because my life is on the line, I get three.

Dr. Peter Dottino, director of gynecological oncology at Mount Sinai (now in private practice), tells me that among the fourteen patients they have treated with their own high-dose program, there have been six recurrences and one death. The patient who died was a 29-year-old woman; the recurrences were within eight to ten months. (As of this writing, the number of recurrences, says Dottino, has risen to twelve.) When you're subjecting a patient to that sort of toxicity and getting those results, you have to rethink the treatment, Dottino says. He recommends the older interperitoneal wash with systemic intravenous chemotherapy.

Dr. Albert Diesseroth, chief of medical oncology at Yale University, does not believe one or two powerful hits is the way to deal with ovarian cancer.

Ovarian cells are "predominantly quiescent," he says in a phone conversation; they divide every so often, but they don't divide quickly enough to be sensitive to one high dose. Memorial's method of administering Taxol in fifteen weekly doses he finds "intriguing." It would provide "continuous sequentious exposure to the therapy."

"I think at this point in time, that's probably preferable to a few big blasts," he says. "The toxicity and risk is substantial, the effect on your immune system is substantial, and we're not totally sure we can kill all the cells."

The most important opinion for me, because he knows me best and because I know him, is Larry Norton's. He has, it turns out, helped develop this high-dose treatment with David Fennelly, but right now, he does not believe it is for me.

"You had a moderately good tumor at the start," Norton says. "Not the very best, but good. Second-look showed you did well with chemotherapy. Not ideal but nowhere near the worst. Disease was minimal. You could be cured now. Your immune system could knock out anything that's left. The advantage of belly wash is, it's been around a long time and it has a long track record. Taxol is very effective. If it doesn't work, if it comes back in a year or two, our knowledge about high-dose will have grown, and we can do it then. You've had two chemotherapies in five years; your bone-marrow recovery might be poor. I would not like you to have a fatal result."

In June, I begin the second round of chemo.

I'm told it should be easier. My dose of Taxol, given weekly, will be 80 milligrams per meter squared instead of 175.

The Cisplatin dosage will be the same, but concentrated in the abdominal cavity, so the side effects will be milder. I will not have to spend the night in the hospital. The doctors tell me I will lose very little hair.

My hair is very important to me—my return to normalcy. It is now just like George Clooney's. In the Village, it is very chic. I've lost ten pounds with surgery. I have my little red convertible. I've gotten much better at the Live-in-the-Moment Number. If the future is unknown, I decide, I will have the best summer of my life: I'll take out the little red car and listen to sixties girl songs and park with guys off the Belt Parkway, just like I did when I was at NYU. I'm not gonna be selective, either. Summer of Love Redux.

"Cancer makes me wild," I tell Herb.

I have my first round of the new chemo in bed in a hospital room. The intravenous Taxol takes an hour this time, and the Benadryl, as usual, leaves me stoned and mellow.

Then the chemo nurse puts a needle into the mediport that makes a lump under the skin just below my ribs. She connects it to a clear two-quart bag of Cisplatin mixed with a saline solution. The infusion takes about two hours. In order to fill up the belly and hit every wrinkle in the abdomen, the Cisplatin is followed by two more liters of saline. I'm told to change positions in order to slosh the drug around.

I cannot feel the Cisplatin as it first goes into my abdomen, but with the second bag of saline, I see my stomach stretch, and I can feel it. By the next morning, I feel normal.

But once again, life with chemo doesn't go as planned.

Three weeks after starting treatment, my hair starts falling out. Since I get Taxol weekly, I have to take steroids weekly. There is a condition, related to heavy steroid use, called Cushing's Syndrome. I get it. My face, just as described in the literature, becomes "round, red, and full"; I have what is described as "trunkal obesity"—my midriff becomes thick and suety. I have put on weight in my life, but no matter how much I gained, I had a waist. Now, I am beginning to be lost to myself. Steroids also give me a hump at the base of my neck. It's temporary, the doctors tell me. It is hard to consider yourself a major babe with a hump. It's more, with the heavy makeup, like the Pillsbury Doughboy's Divorcée Sister.

But I try.

I buy big, baggy shirts to hide the hump, and panty girdles—the laciest and prettiest I can find—to regain my shape. I get a leopard-skin chiffon scarf to tether my blonde wig to my head and drive the little red car around the Hudson Valley, playing "He's a Rebel" on my very fine sound system, flirting with truck drivers. The Summer of Love thing is not actually working out—I don't feel well at all; my sex drive is nil—but on the road, the girl songs make me romantic, and, just like the Crystals, I dream about it.

In August, I make the four-hour drive to Cambridge, to spend some time with my friend Cheryl, whom Herb and I visited years ago in Africa. Cheryl came to New York to look after me when Herb was away. She has seen me during the first chemotherapy, when I did not have the strength to get off the couch. I remember us driving around the Ngong hills, listening to the Pointer Sisters. It is important to me that we have fun again.

But I am not in great shape. My red-blood-cell count has been steadily dropping; walking in Harvard Square, I gasp for oxygen. Coming home, going to a rest stop on the Massachusetts Turnpike, I catch my reflection in the bathroom mirror and see not a blonde Varga girl in a cute retro scarf but a strangely androgynous person with a thick, masculine body and a moon face. The blonde hair is obviously a wig, and a poor one at that. The face is meaty and red from the summer sun. My flirtations with truck drivers now seem ludicrous and pathetic. When I get back to the city, I hide in my apartment.

In September 1996, I am finished with chemotherapy. My ovarian blood-screen results are splendid. I began treatment with a CA-125 of 20; I ended with a 7.

I go to Weight Watchers and start knocking off the twenty pounds I've gained since this nightmare started and spend a lot of the next two months sleeping.

Then I start looking for answers.

XIII

IT HAD BEEN THE UNDERSTANDING of the
Middle-aged Mutant Writer that, except for her
father's prostate cancer, there is no cancer in the
family. But after I write about having had breast
cancer, in the spring of 1992, I get a letter from a
woman in Chicago that makes me wonder.

The woman's last name is Wadler; she has had
breast cancer, also. Growing up, she was told all the
Wadlers are related. Could we be cousins?

I call the Chicago Wadler and tell her what I
know: The Wadlers are a small Jewish family from
Poland; like her, I, too, had been told all Wadlers
were related. We go back to our grandfathers'
generation, but we don't see a connection: If she is a
cousin, she is very distant.

A short time later, a woman in the audience at a
breast-cancer conference tells me that there is
sometimes a link between fathers with prostate

cancer and daughters with breast cancer. I know this proves nothing: Breast cancer and prostate cancer are both common diseases. Still, it starts me thinking: My father had no sisters, so how would we know if there was breast cancer in the family?

As for my grandfather Jacob Wadler, for whom I am named, I know very little: He had five brothers and one sister. He comes from Poland in 1912, at age 18, and buys a little farm-boardinghouse in the Catskills. He falls in love with my grandmother Gussie Belinsky, a guest, and follows her back to the city, showing up unexpectedly at the factory where she works.

"Dark, like an Italian," says Gram, *Italian* being a euphemism in my family for *hot*. "Good-looking. He came for me at the shop—he was dressed so good, I thought he was a boss."

Jacob Wadler is killed by a falling tree while bringing in the cows during a thunderstorm when he is 48. After his death, my family hears nothing from Jacob's relatives in New York City. My father, who is 19, quits college to support his mother and two younger brothers. Thirty years later, when a Wadler from New York comes to the family's lumberyard in Fleischmanns, wondering if we are cousins, my uncle Artie, a former Marine, throws him out.

"Your father didn't want anything to do with us when my father died, and the hell with you," he says.

I start hearing about "the Jewish gene"—a genetic mutation that puts you at a higher risk for breast and ovarian cancer—around the time I'm diagnosed with ovarian cancer, in the fall of 1995. The mutation has been found in Ashkenazic Jews, Jews of Eastern European descent.

I know right away that I want to be tested for it.

For the most part, it's because I'm enraged. I'm a fairly healthy person; I don't smoke, I exercise, and yet, before age 48, I've had two illnesses that have threatened my life. I want to know why; the fact that I've already had the cancers is irrelevant.

I make an appointment with Karen Brown, a counselor at the genetics department at Memorial, and with Dr. Ken Offit, the chief of cancer-genetic services, who also chairs the genetics subcommittee of the American Society of Clinical Oncology.

Brown and Offit have seen families with three generations of breast and ovarian cancers—with only one first-degree relative with cancer, my family, at first glance, would not seem to be high-risk.

There is something about my history, though, that does suggest I might be carrying one of the Ashkenazic Jewish mutations: The mean age for breast and ovarian cancer in the general population is the late fifties.

Inherited cancers, however, tend to occur early.

Twenty percent of Jewish women diagnosed with breast cancer before age 41 have been found to be carrying a mutation. The mean age for ovarian cancer, in that population, is 48. I was diagnosed with breast cancer just after my 43rd birthday and with ovarian cancer at 47—as a possible carrier, I'm right on target.

Karen starts explaining genetics.

I know as soon as she shows me the pictures of paired chromosomes that I prefer Herb's version, which he has been doing ever since I told him I was going for testing.

"It all began vit Gregor Mendel. 'Dese are dah Jewish peas, and dese are dah Gentile peas . . .' "

But I'm determined to make science my friend, so I concentrate:

"BRCA1 and BRCA2 are genes that control cell growth and division. . . . If there is a mutation, it increases the possibility that cancer will develop. . . . Both men and women can inherit the mutation. . . . There is a specific mutation of the BRCA1 gene called 185delAG and a mutation of the BRCA2 gene called 6174delT which seems to be common among

Ashkenazic Jews. It is estimated that one in 50 Ashkenazic Jews carries one of those genes."

The biggest risk for carriers of a BRCA mutation is breast cancer. There's a 66 to 85 percent risk of developing the disease by age 70. Men with the mutation have a 7 percent higher risk than the rest of the population of developing prostate cancer. (Aha! That could explain my father's cancer!) All carriers may have a slightly increased risk of colon cancer. The risk for ovarian cancer is far less clear: Various studies have reported it from 10 to 80 percent, a range so wide I consider it worthless.

(A National Institute of Health study released since this meeting estimates that one in 40 Ashkenazic Jews carries a BRCA mutation. That report cited a breast-cancer risk of 56 percent and a 16 percent risk of ovarian and prostate cancer.)

These are all clearly diseases where knowing your genetic predisposition can save your life. Women carrying the gene are advised to have mammograms and breast exams earlier than the general population, at age 35—even as early as age 25. Protecting yourself against ovarian cancer, according to a department information sheet, is "more difficult."

"Women may participate in research, that is, looking at ultrasound to see if this test, together with pelvic examination and certain blood tests, can help find ovarian cancer early," the fact sheet says. "[They] can also have their ovaries removed to try to prevent ovarian cancer."

Genetic testing is still very new; it takes two months to get the results. I don't worry. Unless the mutations also carry the risk of late marriage, I've had almost everything you can get. Then, in late November, just one day before I'm to go to the hospital to get my test results, there's news. According to a study of ovarian-cancer patients at the University of Pennsylvania, women who carry the BRCA1 mutation have a survival advantage, living twice as long as women without the gene—an average of 77 months.

I get out my calculator and crunch the numbers, the way I used to figure royalties: 77 months equals 6.4 years minus 1 year since diagnosis . . . 5.4 years! And that doesn't factor in Taxol the Wonder Drug!

Reality, once again, is more fantastic than anything Herb and I could ever come up with. I go to my appointment with Karen Brown and Ken Offit praying I have a genetic predisposition for cancer.

And this time—oh, lucky me; I must be, after all, the luckiest of downtown writers—I get what I want: I am carrying the 185delAG mutation.

I call the Chicago Wadler. I'm a little concerned about this; I don't want anyone to panic.

She reacts just the way I'd hoped.

"Thank you," she says.

Then I start nosing around the family, tracking second cousins I haven't spoken to for 20 and 30 years.

Turns out, there *is* cancer. In addition to my grandmother Wadler's sister, Frieda, who died of pancreatic cancer in her fifties, my grandmother had a niece named Eve who's had three cancers: uterine at age 55, breast at 62, and thyroid at 72.

"In our family, there was no cancer, except your father had it," Eve says. "Oh, wait a minute, my mother, Sarah—your grandmother Gussie's sister—had it! Uterine! She didn't die of it; she died a year later from asthma. How could I forget that?"

I don't know that, genetically, this is important. Cancer is the second-leading cause of death in the country. Uterine cancer is not known to be carried on the 185delAG mutation. But it's more cancer than I knew existed in the family.

I move to my grandfather Jacob Wadler's family, the ones I now think of as the lost tribes.

Two Wadlers are listed in the old Manhattan phone book I use to prop up my computer, and, my grandmother would be happy to see, one is a lawyer and one is a doctor. Neither believes we are closely related (though one will turn out to be wrong). Neither has cancer in the family. They direct me on a Wadler chase around town. I don't learn anything about cancer, but since we share the same name, they've noticed my byline over the years: Everyone asks about my health and whether I ever got married.

I trot back to my primary source, the Chicago Wadler. Her mother, the genealogical expert, comes to the phone to explain: There are two branches of Wadlers, Ours and The Cousins. It's hard to sort them out; because Ours often married Cousins, they were "gnipped and gbendeled"—all mixed up.

I check the Gilda Radner Familial Ovarian Cancer Registry outside Buffalo: no Wadlers.

I check an online phone directory: 146 Wadlers.

Then I get lucky: A cousin turns up a phone number for Estelle Essler, the daughter of my grandfather's only sister, Hensche.

Cancer in the family?

Definitely, Estelle says. She had uterine cancer years ago; her sister died of pancreatic cancer. Another cousin knows more. My grandfather did not have one sister; he had *four* sisters. One, Edith Wadler, who moved to Chicago, died of breast cancer. Two never left Poland. They died with their families in the Holocaust.

I am on a two-part mission here: to find out whether there is cancer in the family and to find Wadlers who are related to me and let them know they have a cousin who is carrying a genetic mutation, so that they can protect themselves. Hearing my grandfather had sisters who were murdered by Hitler is not something I expected.

"Everybody was killed?" I ask.

No, the cousin says. Two got out. A few days later, I am speaking with my father's first cousin, who is 70. The Wadlers? A very important family, he says. In Poland, in the city of Szczucin, there was a street that was all Wadlers. Cancer? As a matter of fact, he had colon cancer four years ago, when he was 64. Two years ago, they found cancer in his liver, but now, *kineahora,* he feels great.

Cancer in the Wadler family? His cousin, Sachie, the other one who got out, had uterine cancer. But in general, the Wadlers were healthy, except for his grandmother, who died early—he doesn't know of what. In Europe then, a lot of the time you didn't know why somebody died.

" 'The *teivel uht im ganimin'*—'The devil took him,' " they would say.

And my cousin was very young.

"When Hitler came into Poland, I was 11; I had my bar mitzvah in the bunker," he says. "The camp I was in was called Mielec. It was an airplane factory for Aerosmit; the woman I married later on was there. We would talk to each other through the barbed wire. . . . My daughter is 50; a beautiful, good-looking blonde lady. She has four children. . . ."

The beautiful good-looking blonde lady, from what I'm hearing, may be at risk for cancer. I start to tell the new cousin my medical history. He interrupts, misunderstanding.

"Okay, Joyce, but don't be upset," he says. "God is good, we beat it. Let's hope we'll be okay."

I get off the phone and go into the living room, to Herb.

"I don't get this at all," I say. "I just had a conversation with a guy who lost almost his whole family in the Holocaust, and had a cancer that went to his liver, and he's telling me not only there is a God, but God is good."

Ultimately, excluding my father's prostate cancer and my own cancers, I discover two cases of breast cancer, four of uterine, two of pancreatic, one of colon, and one of thyroid on my father's side of the family I also learn that three of my cousins, making a run to the railroad station during the German occupation of Poland, were identified as Jews and were stoned to death with bricks by the Poles. I am unable to find any other case of ovarian cancer in the family.

XIV

SPEAKING WITH A SOCIAL worker at memorial
Sloan-Kettering who had once worked with an
ovarian-cancer support group, the Mutant hears a
terrifying story: Of 24 women in that group, 18 had
originally been misdiagnosed. But the diagnosis I
most wonder about is my own; is there any way my
cancer could have been caught earlier?

My doctors, as well as ovarian patients I've
spoken with, say the CA-125 tests are flawed,
particularly in premenopausal women. They pick up
many noncancerous conditions: fibroids,
endometriosis, cysts, peritonitis. All can register as
false positives. They miss 50 percent of Stage One
cancers. Test results can be elevated in women who
are perfectly healthy. The sonogram also has both
false positives and false negatives, subjecting women
to unnecessary surgery.

I think the tests have a lot to offer:

A breast-cancer blood screen saved—or at least extended—my life. I believe that if I'd been followed with the ovarian blood test, the cancer would have been found even earlier. True, the sonogram in my case did not reflect the extent of the disease, but it certainly indicated cancer. It showed bilateral solid masses, fluid at the base of the pelvis, blood flow. If the tests on their own are unreliable, why not screen with both of them, as a check-and-balance system?

The tests aren't cheap, but they aren't prohibitive: The CA-125 blood test, at Memorial, costs the patient $92; a sonogram is $328. In a study at the University of Kentucky Medical Center I find, in which sonograms were provided free, the hospital got the cost of a sonogram to under $25. "Expenses compare favorably with diagnostic procedures for other diseases," the report says.

There are twice as many cases of ovarian cancer a year as cervical cancer; ovarian cancer kills more women than all the other gynecological cancers combined. I've had Pap smears, the test for cervical cancer, since I was 18. Approaching the age when ovarian cancer occurs, I was never told about sonograms—even with my history of breast cancer.

I call up my original doctor, the gynecologist who writes books, whom I have not heard from since tests indicated cancer. I had a sonogram before I was diagnosed that seemed pretty effective, I tell him when he gets back to me. Since I'd had unusual bleeding, why hadn't a sonogram ever been used to check me out?

It sounds like he has my records in front of him: Bleeding is not considered a sign of ovarian cancer he tells me; it's a sign of endometrial cancer. He checked for that in November 1995. But I had a history of breast cancer, I say, and since women with breast cancer are supposed to have a higher risk of ovarian—

He interrupts, taking the question away from me. "You raise a good question," he says. "Should every woman have a routine vaginal sonogram—"

"Not every woman," I say, though that interests me also. "Women with a history of breast cancer."

He keeps talking.

"No one has ever done it routinely," he says. "There's a question of cost-effectiveness. It's like the whole thing about mammograms for women between 40 and 50."

The cost of the endometrial biopsy I had in his office was $600, I tell him. Sonograms are much cheaper.

"If you have bleeding from the uterus, you check out the uterus," he says. "Look, I've got a roomful of patients, I've got to go. It sounds like you're holding your own."

I'm left without an answer. Then I remember something. The book-writing gynecologist once gave me one of his books. If it survived the medical-book purge of over a year ago, it's in the house.

I find the section on gynecological cancers.

"Women with a family history of breast cancer, colon cancer, ovarian cancer or uterine cancer need to be carefully screened for ovarian cancer," the gynecologist has written. "Screening the entire population has not been shown to be cost-effective or to change the survival rate. However, in women with a family history as noted, twice-yearly pelvic examinations, blood tests (known as CA-125) and pelvic sonograms should be done."

I collapse on the floor near the bookshelves, furious and sobbing. Doesn't having had breast cancer put you in the category of women "with a family history"? Am I going to die because a doctor didn't follow his own screening advice?

I reread the section. *Family history.* It's actually rather ambiguous. In a court of law, one might argue it refers to hereditary cancers. Might the doctor believe having a mother or a sister who has had cancer somehow puts you more at risk than having had cancer yourself?

I doubt it. I also doubt that I could get a direct answer from the doctor at this point.

I track down an expert: Dr. Arthur C. Fleischer, head of diagnostic sonography at Vanderbilt University, co-author of *Early Detection of Ovarian Cancer With Transvaginal Sonography: Potentials and Limitations* and thirteen other books in the field.

How effective is sonography in picking up ovarian cancer?

"Very effective," Dr. Fleischer says. "We did a study evaluating 206 patients who were at risk and found 27 cancers over a seven-year period—70 percent with Stage One. So we can find them very early."

And why were those patients considered to be at risk?

"Either a history of breast, colon, or endometrial cancer," the doctor says.

So if you'd had breast cancer, you'd be considered at risk?

"Oh, yeah. Definitely," Dr. Fleischer says.

I make an appointment with Larry Norton. "I know you saved my life with that blood screen," I say, "and thank you."

"Oh you're welcome," he says.

"But the question that keeps tormenting me," I say, "is why, in the best cancer hospital in the country, I had a cancer that wasn't found until it was a Stage Three."

"Because you had bad luck," Norton says.

I feel like my dead grandmother, who talked to me in Yiddish and told me I should only be lucky, is in the room.

This is the guy who writes about the growth curve of tumors and sits on the editorial boards of five professional journals and is famous for some carcino-mathematical mumbo-jumbo called the Norton-Simon Hypothesis, which he happily tells me I could not understand in a million years, and I agree. Now he's telling me it all comes down to luck?

"That's right," says Norton. "I did the most sensitive tests we could do—the breast-cancer screen, the CEA screen. You just had the bad fortune to have a disease that tended to grow in an unusual pattern. Stage Three means it's out of the ovary; typically, it will grow more inside the ovary before it starts to spread out. It couldn't have been there too long, because I was doing blood tests on you and they were never abnormal. *Never.*"

But wouldn't a sonogram have picked it up sooner?

"Probably." Norton says. "It's not very sensitive or specific, but in your case it probably would have. But we had no reason to screen you at the time. You didn't come in with a whole breast-and-ovarian family history. Now, in retrospect, Ashkenazic Jews should be screened carefully. Before, this whole idea was very fuzzy. You were really right at the cusp of an explosion of knowledge."

What about the theory that all women with breast cancer have a higher risk of ovarian cancer and should be regularly screened?

"It wouldn't make sense," Norton says. "Only 10 percent of breast cancers are considered familial; they're the ones with a higher risk of ovarian cancer. And of that 10 percent, maybe you'll be able to catch one or 2 percent with screening. In pre-BRCA1 days, you'd read that people with breast cancer had a higher risk of ovarian cancer, but we didn't know who those people were. Now we can identify a subset.

"It's possible there are mutations that cluster around other groups—we suspect that—but right now, in the New York City area, Ashkenazic Jews are the most numerous population that seem to have this situation. If you are an Ashkenazic Jew with fairly young breast cancer, say under 40, we would indeed talk to you about genetic testing."

Does this mean if you're a Gentile you won't be followed as carefully?

"Of course not," says Norton. "If it's early-onset breast cancer with a Gentile woman or if it's a Sephardic Jew with bilateral breast cancer and a mother with breast cancer, I would think they would be at high risk and should be screened. The whole international community of genetic experts is working on criteria for screening. For now, at Memorial, if a woman comes in with breast cancer and she has a family history, we recommend talking to a genetic counselor. If a woman is carrying the BRCA1 or 2 mutation, we follow them till age 45 with the sonogram and blood test. Then, at age 45, I would counsel them about having their ovaries removed."

He thinks the tests for ovarian cancer are that weak?

"I don't want what happened to you to happen to other people," Norton says. "If you have a population that's very high-risk, and you don't have sensitive ways of diagnosing it, removing the ovaries is your only alternative. It's a terrible alternative, but it's the best we have until we have a better one, which we're working on right now."

We talk for a bit about the tests for ovarian cancer, the capabilities of which we disagree on.

"You know what I think we both missed?" I tell him. "The constipation. I had very intense constipation for two years. I know you and Barakat don't believe I had enough disease to cause it, but I'll go down believing it was a symptom."

"You're wrong," Norton says. "It's magical thinking. You associate the two things because they happened at the same time. And I'm not gonna let you go down."

XV

So **THERE IT IS,** my ovarian adventure. I would like to say it is over, but it is not. I go every three months for examinations and blood tests; my last blood test, eleven months after chemotherapy, was a 6. With any number under 35 considered normal, it doesn't get much better than a 6.

"Does this mean anything, that eleven months out I'm clean?" I ask Barakat hopefully "Is there, like, a curve? Does it maybe take me out of that 50 percent four-year-survival thing?"

I have for some reason become fond of his inability to sugarcoat.

"No," he says. "What is important is if you get to two years, as I'm sure you will, then we take a deep breath. When we hit five years, we pop a huge bottle of Dom Pérignon."

I am ahead of him: I switched from wine to champagne with my first cancer. And when it comes to the Living-in-the-Moment Number, I am a champ. I put the top down on the little red car when it's 50 degrees. I drag people to tango lessons at Lincoln Center. When I hear of a party, I go.

Which is not to say I never get the terrors.

A week before my blood tests, I am so scared I need a pill every night. Going to the Jefferson library in the Village, looking up a *New York Times* piece about a woman dying of ovarian cancer, the Middle-aged Mutant read the entire piece for the first time and got very scared.

The doctors, in that story, said a woman had a one-in-seven chance of surviving ovarian cancer.

The Mutant crunched the numbers, as she tends to do: Diagnosed in 1993; too early for Taxol. And these days, five-year survival for a woman with distant metastases, according to the American Cancer Society, is 25 percent.

Even so, it is not a happy statistic. The Mutant walks out onto Sixth Avenue with her stomach as tight as a fist. She feels like she is going to cry.

On the other hand, it is summer. I have red curly hair. I have Herb. I have a car that whirls with me down the mountains, trailing music. The doctors are right. If I worry, the cancer wins.

I focus: Not on how I will improve my life or find a boyfriend or write the novel that is beginning to form in my head, but on the moment.

It is 5:30 Friday afternoon in Greenwich Village in August. In the world as it is—not the world of the movies, or sixties girl songs—what can I do to extract the most pleasure from the rest of the day?

I think about it. What I want to do, I decide, is to go to a movie with the person I love most and eat ice cream for dinner. And I call up Herb and we do. And I am happy.

Afterword

Protecting Yourself

OVARIAN CANCER IS often called the silent killer. That description infuriates me. I don't think ovarian cancer is silent, I think we haven't been educated enough about the warning signs which, unfortunately, often do not present until a cancer is advanced. But there are still levels of advanced cancer and your chances are much better catching a cancer at a level 3 than a level 4. I also believe that there are steps which can be taken to catch ovarian cancer, which consumers and doctors are not utilizing.

What are possible warning signs of ovarian cancer?

According to the Ovarian Cancer Research Fund warning signs may include abdominal bloating or pain, digestive problems such as constipation and diarrhea, and an increased frequency of urination. Unfortunately, as the group notes, these symptoms can also be indicative of any number of conditions. If they continue for more than two weeks, however, it is recommended you see your doctor and be "a forceful advocate" for yourself.

What does "forceful advocate" mean?

To me, it's demanding answers rather than adapting a wait and see approach. If your GP cannot determine what is causing your medical problems, see your gynecologist and say you want a vaginal sonogram. As a woman doctor wrote to me after I had written about my ovarian cancer experience in New York Magazine in 1997, gynecologists have the equipment to do this test in their offices—they use vaginal sonograms as a matter of routine with pregnant women. In fact, this doctor felt vaginal sonograms should be a part of a woman's annual examination, much like Pap smears. It makes sense to me.

Another important thing every woman should do is to learn about her family's medical history. This is not always easy. In our grandparents' time the word *cancer* was often whispered. The patients themselves often did not know the origin of a gynecological cancer—it was often not diagnosed until it had spread throughout the abdomen or it was described simply as "down there."

If you find multiple cases of breast and ovarian cancer in your family, particularly early onset cancers occurring before the women were in their early 40's, make your doctor aware of it.

According to the American Society of Clinical Oncology the majority of ovarian cancers, about 85%, are not inherited. And having a genetic mutation does not mean that you will develop breast or ovarian cancer.

But it certainly increases the risk.

According to The National Cancer Institute, women who carry the BRCA-1 or BRCA-2 mutation have a 15% to 50% risk of developing ovarian cancer in their lifetime. The risk for women who do not carry the mutation is 1.4%.

The mutation I carry, BRCA-1, has been found in Jewish women of Ashkenazic or Eastern European descent, as has the BRCA-2 gene. When I wrote these stories about my ovarian cancer for New York Magazine, some readers felt there was nothing to be gained by knowing if you carried the gene.

They were wrong.

Knowing that you have a genetic predisposition to ovarian cancer enables you to takes steps which may prevent ovarian cancer or catch it early. You may decide to have your ovaries removed when you know you no longer wish to have children. You may decide to be followed with the CA-125 blood test in combination with a pelvic sonogram. You will certainly be more alert to the symptoms mentioned above and so will your doctor.

Finally—and I cannot stress this enough—if you are diagnosed with ovarian cancer go to a National Cancer Institute designated cancer center to discuss treatment, even if you cannot have your treatment there—they will be aware of the newest drugs and treatments and your local hospital and doctors may be able to follow their recommendations. I've included a link below. And make sure your surgery is performed by a gynecologic oncologist, not a general surgeon. The more cancer the surgeon can remove, the better your chance of survival.

Most of all remember that cancer is not a death sentence—but it is an illness in which the decisions you make may save your life. Get your information from cancer care professionals, not the friends and family members who suddenly decide they are experts; take a friend with you to take notes or record the conversations; get second and third opinions; and make sure you are getting the best treatment available.

Helpful Links

To find a National Cancer Institute Cancer centers near you go to:
www.cancer.gov/researchandfunding/extramural/
      cancercenters.

For information about ovarian cancer detection and treatment, go to the Ovarian Cancer Research Fund web site:
www.ocrf.org.

Detailed information on the genetics of ovarian cancer can be found at:
www.cancer.gov/cancertopics/pdq/genetics/breast-
      and-ovarian/HealthProfessional.

SHARE, a self-help group for women with breast and ovarian cancer, provides information as well as support.
http://www.sharecancersupport.org/share-new.

About the Author

JOYCE **WADLER** is a New York City humorist who writes the "I Was Misinformed" column for *The New York Times,* where she was a staff reporter for 15 years.

Before coming to the *Times,* Ms. Wadler worked as a feature writer and crime reporter for newspapers and magazines. She was the New York correspondent for *The Washington Post* as well as a contributing writer for *New York* Magazine and *Rolling Stone.*

Her books include *My Breast,* her memoir about breast cancer, which she later adapted as a CBS television movie; and *Liaison,* the story of the French civil servant and the Chinese opera singer which inspired the play *M. Butterfly.*

An E-QUALITY PRESS Book

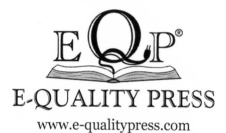

E-QUALITY PRESS
www.e-qualitypress.com